Neonatal Neurology
Fourth Edition

Editor: Susan Pioli
Developmental Editor: Joan Ryan
Project Manager: Glenys Norquay
Designer: Stewart Larking
Marketing Manager: Matthew Latuchie

Neonatal Neurology

Fourth Edition

Edited by

Gerald M. Fenichel, M.D.
Professor of Neurology and Pediatrics
Chief, Division of Pediatric Neurology
Vanderbilt University School of Medicine
Neurologist-in Chief
The Monroe Carell Jr. Children's Hospital at Vanderbilt
Nashville, Tennessee

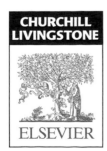

CHURCHILL
LIVINGSTONE

ELSEVIER

CHURCHILL
LIVINGSTONE
ELSEVIER
An imprint of Elsevier Inc.

First edition 1980
Second edition 1985
Third edition 1990

ISBN-13: 978 0 443 06724 2
ISBN-10: 0 443 06724 4

British Library Cataloguing in Publication Data
A catalogue record for this book is available from the British Library

Library of Congress Cataloging in Publication Data
A catalog record for this book is available from the Library of Congress

Notice
Medical knowledge is constantly changing. Standard safety precautions must be followed, but as new research and clinical experience broaden our knowledge, changes in treatment and drug therapy may become necessary or appropriate. Readers are advised to check the most current product information provided by the manufacturer of each drug to be administered to verify the recommended dose, the method and duration of administration, and contraindications. It is the responsibility of the practitioner, relying on experience and knowledge of the patient, to determine dosages and the best treatment for each individual patient. Neither the Publisher nor the authors assume any liability for any injury and/or damage to persons or property arising from this publication.

The Publisher

Printed in China

Last digit is the print number: 9 8 7 6 5 4 3 2 1

CONTENTS

CONTRIBUTING AUTHORS

Gregory N. Barnes, M.D., Ph.D.
Associate Professor of Neurology and Pediatrics, Division of Pediatric
Neurology, Vanderbilt University School of Medicine, Nashville, Tennessee

Gerald M. Fenichel, M.D.
Professor of Neurology and Pediatrics; Chief, Division of Pediatric Neurology,
Vanderbilt University School of Medicine; Neurologist-in Chief, The Monroe
Carell Jr. Children's Hospital at Vanderbilt, Nashville, Tennessee

Alan Hill, M.D., Ph.D.
Professor and Head, Division of Neurology, British Columbia Children's
Hospital, Vancouver, Canada

Joseph J. Nania, M.D.
Assistant Professor of Pediatrics, Division of Pediatric Infectious Diseases,
Vanderbilt University School of Medicine; Attending Pediatrician,
The Monroe Carell Jr. Children's Hospital at Vanderbilt, Nashville, Tennessee

Elke H. Roland, M.D.
Associate Professor, Division of Neurology, University of British Columbia;
Pediatric Neurologist, British Columbia Children's Hospital, Vancouver,
Canada

Jörn-Hendrik Weitkamp, M.D.
Fellow, Division of Neonatology, Vanderbilt University School of Medicine;
Attending Pediatrician, The Monroe Carell Jr. Children's Hospital at
Vanderbilt, Nashville, Tennessee

PREFACE

Publication of the third edition of *Neonatal Neurology* was in 1990. Its intention was to 'serve as a readable guide for clinicians, not as a comprehensive reference.' Such a need still exists; therefore a fourth edition. The field has expanded greatly with the development and expansion of neonatal intensive care. I could no longer manage the field alone, and therefore invited experts to contribute.

The general chapter format remains the same, but some sections have been expanded considerably in recognition of advances in those fields. For these, I have asked others to contribute. For the discussion of genetic disorders, I rely greatly on internet sources such as *Online Mendelian Inheritance in Man* and *GeneClinics*. Having recently published the fifth edition of *Clinical Pediatric Neurology*, I used portions of that text appropriate for this volume.

Gerald M. Fenichel, M.D.
Nashville, 2006

1
The Neurological Consultation
Gerald M. Fenichel

Seizures, hypotonia, and states of decreased responsiveness are the clinical features that most often prompt neurological consultation. Often, the neurologist comes on the scene long after the acute event is over to answer questions concerning prognosis and to serve as the future health provider for chronic care. The approach to neurological consultation in the newborn is the same as in older children. The neurologist must provide a diagnosis, assess current neurological status, recommend treatment options, and define prognosis. The last is often uncertain. Newborns have remarkable resiliency, and morphology, as displayed on brain imaging, does not always precisely predict later function.

Diagnostic accuracy has improved considerably with the introduction of techniques that image the brain: computed tomography (CT), ultrasound scanning (US), and magnetic resonance imaging (MRI). It is now commonplace to know what has happened to the nervous system, the greater difficulty is to know why it happened. The birth of an imperfect child generates guilt and self-defensiveness in the parents and in the doctors involved. One feels an inherent need to determine specific fault, but in many situations, the identification of a single event as etiological in the evolution of a brain damage syndrome is impossible.

The assessment of neurological status usually provides adequate information to localize abnormalities in the central and peripheral nervous system and determine severity. Such an assessment serves three purposes. The first is rapid diagnosis of a fixed deficit or syndrome; the second is the development a differential diagnosis that laboratory tests or time will further clarify; and the third is to provide a baseline examination in the continuing evaluation of the child.

Treatment recommendations and prognostic expectations are related. Long-term outcome is clear in occasional situations, but more often, we deal with children who are 'at risk,' and estimates of the degree of risk are imprecise. The only practical link between treatment and long-term prognosis concerns decisions on the continuation or removal of life-support systems. When this is

1

not an issue, the focus of attention should be on prompt medical intervention. Accomplishing the latter is only by the anticipation of problems through knowledge of the natural course of the disease process.

TERMINOLOGY

The terminology used for the developmental periods during and following pregnancy are derived in part from common usage and in part from health organization definitions for the reporting of mortality statistics. This text uses the following terms:

Fetus: A fetus is a developing child from the time of conception to the time of delivery. From conception to 12 weeks' gestation, the fetus is an embryo, because organogenesis is incomplete; this division is an arbitrary point in the continuity of development.
Neonate or newborn: A child during the first 28 days after birth.
Infant: A child from 29 days after birth to one year.
Gestational age: The age of the newborn in weeks from time of conception.
Conceptional age: The age of the newborn in weeks from time of conception; gestational age plus postpartum age.
Perinatal: The period from 20 weeks' gestation to 28 days after birth.
Antepartum or prenatal: The period from conception to the onset of labor.
Intrapartum: During labor.
Postpartum or postnatal: After delivery.
Prematurity: Birth prior to 36 weeks' gestational age and at a birth weight of less than 2500 g.

HISTORICAL EVENTS

Most historical information is not first-hand, but derived from the notes of others. In newborns transported to an intensive care nursery from other hospitals, and even in newborns born in the same hospital, the available data concerning antepartum care and delivery are often incomplete. Logic exists in compiling the clinical history in chronological order. Begin with the genetic and social factors that preceded pregnancy, continue with the quality and duration of antepartum care and the circumstances of labor and delivery, and conclude with the management of the newborn in the immediate and critical first hours after delivery.

Gestational Age

An accurate estimate of gestational age is important to address the questions of etiology, diagnosis, treatment, and prognosis. A pediatrician or neonatologist usually assesses gestational age, but the neurologist must review the data supporting the estimate. Sources of information for gestational dating derive from several sources: the mother's report of the last normal menstrual period, the physical appearance, and neurological assessment of the newborn, and measurements of intrauterine growth and weight. The physical signs of maturity are the most reliable guides to gestational age (Amiel-Tison et al., 1999). The date of the last menstrual period may not be available, or may be in error due to post-conceptional bleeding or the use of birth control pills. Neurological maturity is difficult to judge in a child who is not neurologically normal, and intrauterine disease may unfavorably alter intrauterine growth. However, a strong correlation among physical examination, menstrual history, and the percentiles for intrauterine growth permits the greatest degree of confidence in the accuracy of gestational dating.

Preconceptional Events

Significant forces that influence the outcome of pregnancy are already at work before conception. Expression of the defect in one or both parents or if a previous pregnancy has produced a similarly affected child suggests a genetic defect. In the absence of these clues, the physician must gather information concerning the possibilities of consanguinity of the parents and genetic disorders in other relatives. Abortion and stillbirth experiences in the parent's families require determination. The information is difficult to elicit and often delivered in small parcels over time, surfacing as resistance erodes to sharing family secrets with a stranger. It is also common for the child's parents to be genuinely unaware that family members with genetic disorders exist in one or both pedigrees. Preceding generations never shared the information with the next generation.

The health, attitudes, and resources of the mother prior to conception determine the environment for fertilization of the egg and are of no less importance than genetic factors in the development of the fetus. Social and economic deprivations that are present prior to conception are likely to have a continuing effect on the fetus during pregnancy.

Make specific inquiries into the state of maternal health: especially the presence of diabetes, infection, and toxemia; exposure to drugs and alcohol; and evidence of placental dysfunction. With the exception of maternal drug use and certain specific syndromes of the newborn (rubella, infant of a diabetic mother), the establishment of a causal relationship between antepartum events and pregnancy outcome is fraught with uncertainty.

Intrapartum History

The time from the onset of labor to delivery is the period of greatest vulnerability of the fetus to infection and asphyxia. However, the results of the Collaborative Perinatal Study as reported by Nelson and collaborators in a series of papers highlighted the difficulty in relating specific events during labor and delivery and outcome. An established association does not exist between specific obstetrical complication and a bad neurological outcome in term newborns. Cerebral palsy occurs in only 2% of surviving newborns whose fetal heart rate had been less than 60 per minute. In a prospective study of almost 3000 labors and deliveries, the incidence of meconium staining of the amniotic fluid was 22%. However, only 0.4% of term newborns with meconium-stained amniotic fluid later showed cerebral palsy.

Postpartum History

The height, weight, and head circumference at birth as expected for gestational age give some indication of the quality of intrauterine life, while the Apgar scores and blood gases provide information on the condition of the child at birth. However, most newborns with low 5-minute Apgar scores will be neurologically normal and a blood pH of 7.0 or greater does not correlate with outcome. The need for prolonged resuscitation, altered states of consciousness, seizures, deficient movement, and disturbances at sucking and swallowing are all significant historical events pointing to neurological dysfunction during the postpartum period.

The intent of the Apgar scoring system was to grade the health of term newborns and not premature newborns. Indeed, premature newborns rarely survived when Dr Apgar created the scale.

The timing and sequence of events are important clues to diagnosis. The probable cause of seizures on the first day postpartum is quite different from the probable cause of seizures on the fourth or seventh days (see Table 2–2).

CLINICAL EXAMINATION

This section describes a method of physical examination for the purpose of clinical diagnosis. It does not constitute everything possible to test, but only those tests required for rapid clinical assessment and diagnosis in the nursery. The sequence of the examination is important. The method of examination requires little modification when testing relatively healthy newborns whose gestational ages vary from 30 to 40 weeks, although the responses obtained vary markedly, but predictably, at different stages of maturity (Table 1–1). As a rule, handle premature newborns as little as possible and rely more on observation. Major modifications in technique are required for sick newborns in which mechanical ventilation, hypothermia, and monitoring devices interdict excessive handling of the child.

Inspection at Rest

Most term newborns are asleep, as this state occupies an average 17 hours of the first day. Remove covers carefully without waking the child and allow time for observation. In sleep, the eyes are closed, respiration is regular, and one notes

TABLE 1–1   Neurological maturation

Function	26 Weeks	30 Weeks	34 Weeks	38 Weeks
Resting	Flexion of arms, flexion or extension of legs	Flexion of arms, flexion or extension of legs	Flexion of all limbs	Flexion of all limbs
Arousal	Unable to maintain	Remain briefly	Remain awake	Maintain awake
Rooting	Absent	Long latency	Present	
Sucking	Absent	Long latency	Weak	Vigorous
Pupillary reflex	Absent	Variable	Present	Present
Traction	No response	No response	Head lag	Mild head lag
Moro	No response	Flexion or extension of legs	Flexion or extension of legs	Complete
Withdrawal	Absent	Withdrawal only	Crossed extension	Crossed extension

random movements in all limbs. With an oral feeding tube in place, sucking movements on the tube are common.

The initial observation, made with little physical contact, includes a search for dysmorphic features of the face and hands, malformations, evidence of physical trauma, and the presence of seizures. Extend the time devoted to inspection in newborns with a seizure history. Clinical manifestations of seizures in the newborn are quite different from those encountered later in infancy and childhood and described in detail in Chapter 2.

Pay considerable attention to resting posture, as this is one of the more important clues to neurological health. All normal newborns from 32 to 40 weeks' gestation lie with some degree of abduction at the thighs and flexion at the elbows, hips, and ankles (Fig. 1–1). Newborns delivered from breech positions are sometimes an exception and keep their legs extended. At 25 to 30 weeks' gestation, the arms are in flexion but the legs are in either flexion or extension. Abduction tone in the thighs is present even at 25 weeks' gestation.

Any newborn of 25 weeks' gestation or older who lies with all limbs in full extension should be considered abnormal. The severity of the abnormality relates directly to the maturity of the child. The 'frog-leg' posture, in which abduction of the legs is sufficient to cause the lateral thigh to rest upon the supporting surface, is a definite sign of depressed postural tone. Two positions of the arms are equivalent to the frog-leg posture: flexion at the elbow with the dorsa of the hands against the supporting surface and the upward facing palms beside the head, and flaccid extension (Fig. 1–2). Both indicate depressed postural tone of the arms.

The normal hand, loosely fisted with the thumb outside of the other fingers, may open and close spontaneously during sleep. A tightly fisted hand, with the thumb constantly enclosed by the other fingers and not opening spontaneously (*fisting*), is abnormal and is sometimes a precursor of spasticity.

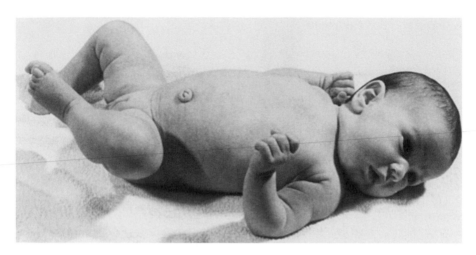

FIGURE 1–1   Normal resting posture. There is adduction of the thighs and an attitude of flexion in the limb joints.

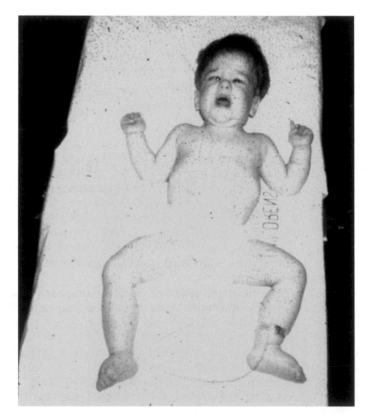

FIGURE 1–2   Abnormal resting posture. The thighs are fully abducted (frog-leg) and the arms lie in a flaccid position beside the head.

Examination of the Head

The first physical contact with the child is gentle palpation of the fontanelles and sutures. Appraising their size and tenseness is impossible in an aroused crying child, and the palpation requires soothing movements of one or two fingers. The anterior fontanelle, at the junction of the coronal, metopic, and sagittal sutures, is the one most commonly used to evaluate intracranial pressure. Its size in normal newborns at all gestational ages is quite variable. The metopic and coronal sutures should not admit a fingertip. Excessive widening of these sutures at birth is more commonly associated with long-standing antepartum disturbances such as hydrocephalus and disorders of ossification than with an acute increase in intracranial pressure during the perinatal period.

The tension in the fontanelle is difficult to quantify by palpation, but assessment is possible as to whether it is soft, full, or bulging. A bulging fontanelle rises above the level of the bone edges and is sufficiently tense to cause difficulty in determining where the bone ends and the fontanelle begins. This condition is normal in the vigorously crying newborn but is always abnormal in the sleeping state. A full fontanelle is clearly distinguished from the surrounding bone edge but, unlike a soft fontanelle, does not depress to the palpating finger. A full fontanelle is not necessarily abnormal. Factors that impair and confuse the assessment are edema of the scalp, excessive molding, subgaleal hemorrhage, and extravasation of intravenous fluids.

Measurement of head circumference is not the next logical step in examination, as this will arouse the child. Defer the measurement until the end of the examination in order to study arousal by a standard stimulus.

Arousal

To produce arousal, gently shake the thorax with your thumb and index finger. This maneuver produces opening of the eyes and/or facial grimacing, crying, and movement of the limbs. Once aroused, term newborns and premature newborns of at least 34 weeks' gestation often remain awake throughout the examination. Newborns of 28 to 33 weeks' gestation have difficulty in maintaining the alert state for long periods. Newborns of 25 to 27 weeks require frequent stimulation to maintain arousal. Inability to provoke at least facial grimacing and movement of the extremities is abnormal and considered evidence for states of decreased consciousness.

The terms used to describe states of decreased consciousness in older children are difficult to apply to newborns. However, some statement should be recorded as to whether the child can be aroused and if arousal can be sustained. Withdrawal of the foot from pain, a spinal reflex, is not an arousal response.

An excessive response to arousal, *jitteriness* (also known as tremulousness), is seen in normal children but is more common in children with encephalopathy and those born to drug dependent mothers (Parker et al., 1990). Low frequency, high-amplitude shaking of the limbs and jaw characterizes the response. A low threshold for the Moro reflex is commonly associated. However, the movements also occur in the absence of any apparent external manipulation and then mistaken for seizures. Distinguish jitteriness from seizures by electroencephalographic (EEG) monitoring and the following clinical criteria: provocation by stimulation, absence of eye movements, and lack of change in respiratory pattern. It commonly accompanies arousal in lethargic or obtunded newborns and can be the only evidence of arousal from the stuporous state.

A *hyperalert state* characterized by full wakefulness and jitteriness for periods up to 18 hours may occur in asphyxiated newborns. The eyes are widely open but lack visual tracking and the Moro reflex is easy to elicit (see Ch. 4).

Cranial Nerves

The grimacing and crying following arousal provide an opportunity to evaluate the fullness of facial expression. The eyes may open briefly, but forced closure of the lids is more common. As the mouth opens in a cry, the corners displace downward, and the nasolabial folds deepen. Observe the tongue and palate when the mouth opens. The quality of the newborn cry and its alteration in certain pathological states is rarely of value in defining neurological status.

Once aroused and disturbed, the child must be soothed and comforted so that the cranial nerve examination can be continued in the alert but quiet state. Providing the opportunity to suck is the initial step. Touching the perioral skin at the corners of the mouth elicits the *rooting response*. The complete response is usually present at 32 weeks' gestation. Turning the head toward the side stimulated, opening the mouth, and grasping of the examiner's fingertip between the lips is characteristic. Rooting is present at 28 weeks' gestation, but the response is slow and incomplete. Even at term, the response is not constant and its absence on a single attempt on the first day postpartum is not abnormal. When rooting is weak or absent, the examiner should insert the tip of the finger into the mouth to test sucking. At 28 to 30 weeks' gestation, the suck is slow, weak, and not sustainable. With each succeeding week of maturity, it becomes more vigorous; by 36 weeks' gestation, the newborn exerts sufficient force to sustain adequate feeding. The rooting and sucking responses test partial functions of cranial nerves V, VII, and XII. The act of swallowing tests cranial nerves IX and X. The brainstem coordinates all three responses.

Only in an unconscious newborn, can the use of force accomplish lid opening. Most newborns open their eyes spontaneously when they begin to suck. This provides the opportunity to test ocular motility. Ocular alignment in the newborn is usually poor. Approximately 2% of newborns exhibit a tendency for chronic downward deviation of the eyes during the waking state. The eyes are in a normal position during sleep and can move upward reflexively. The *doll's eye maneuver* tests reflex eye movements even in premature newborns. The free hand rotates the head gently from side to side, to provoke contralateral eye movements. The pupillary reflex is consistently present after 31 weeks' gestation but is technically difficult to assess because of the *dazzle reflex*, in which a bright light causes immediate and sustained closure of the eyes for as long as the light is present.

Vision and hearing are not clinically assessable, but are testable with evoked responses if there is any question of impairment. The doll's eye maneuver partially assesses the vestibular portion of cranial nerve VIII. The Moro reflex is another method for testing vestibular function. Responses to odors and tastes are of little clinical importance. Tests of cranial nerve XI are part of the motor examination, and ophthalmoscopic examination is the final portion of the examination.

Tone

Tone is the resistance of muscle to stretch. The nervous system distinguishes between two different types of stretch: *phasic* and *postural*. A short duration, high-amplitude stretch is resisted by a phasic mechanism, which responds with an equally brief but forceful contraction. By contrast, a postural mechanism, which provides a long duration, low-amplitude contraction, resists the sustained, low-amplitude stretch imposed by gravity. The distinction is important because tests of phasic and postural tone are separate and vary independently in certain disease states. *Spasticity* is an abnormal sensitivity of phasic tone in which the pull of gravity becomes a sufficient stimulus to activate the phasic mechanism. In infants, *scissoring* on vertical suspension readily demonstrates spasticity. In newborns, the signs of spasticity are more subtle and expressed as persistent fisting with the thumbs inside the fist, resistance to passive movement, and sustained clonus.

Phasic Tone

Resistance of limbs to movement and the activity of the tendon reflexes assess phasic tone. Since flexion attitude predominates in newborns, resistance to extension is usually measured. Minimal resistance, readily overcome by the examiner is a normal response. After fully extending the leg in newborns of 32 weeks' gestation, recoil to the flexed position occurs. The absence of recoil is not absolute evidence of central nervous system dysfunction (CNS), but increased resistance with exaggerated recoil does suggest early spasticity. Decreased resistance to passive extension is a nonspecific finding encountered in newborns with cerebral depression, spinal injuries, disorders of the motor unit, and systemic illness.

Tendon reflexes are the purest example of the phasic tone mechanism. Tapping the tendon imparts a sudden high-amplitude stretch to the muscle that results in a brief but forceful contraction. The patella tendon reflex is the only tendon reflex consistently present at birth; however, it may be difficult to elicit on the first day postpartum and its absence is not abnormal. The biceps tendon reflex and the ankle tendon reflex are at best inconstant and their presence or absence adds little to the clinical assessment.

To test the patella tendon reflex, first place the child's head with the face in the midline or the tonic neck reflex will impose asymmetries: the knee jerk exaggerates on the side to which the head is turned and depressed on the opposite side. Place the knee in a semiflexed position and the tendon tapped briskly with a small reflex hammer. Adult-size reflex hammers decrease the likelihood of obtaining the response and frequently shake the entire leg sufficiently as to obscure the reflex contraction.

The absence of tendon reflexes usually suggests dysfunction in the motor unit but does not exclude cerebral disorders. Newborns with an acute encephalopathy usually have no tendon reflexes for several days postpartum. Eventually the reflexes return and may become exaggerated.

A few beats of ankle clonus may be present in normal newborns, but sustained clonus is abnormal. The activation of clonus requires a constant state of stretch in the muscle. This is difficult to accomplish by violent dorsiflexion of the foot and the better method is stretching the tendon to a variety of lengths to find the point of excitation for clonus. The preferred technique is to hold the anterior third of the foot with the hip and knee in flexion and then shake it gently as the leg slowly extends. Ankle clonus can be present during an acute encephalopathy when the patella tendon reflex is absent. This indicates that the motor unit is intact.

Postural Tone

Since postural tone is a resistance to the pull of gravity, it is essential at this point in the examination to lift the child from the supine position. Perform three tests of postural tone in sequence: *the traction response, vertical suspension,* and *horizontal suspension.* The traction response is the most sensitive and most useful of the three because it can be tested within the confines of an isolate.

In the healthy mature newborn, initiate the traction response by placing the examiner's index finger in the child's hands to provoke a grasp reflex. The grasp of a healthy term newborn is of sufficient intensity to pull the child almost to a sitting position. However, for testing traction, it is important for the examiner to grasp the child's hands as well. As the child slowly pulls to sitting, the head leaves the surface almost immediately, with only minimal lag behind the body. When attaining the sitting position, the head may continue to lag or may become erect for a moment and then fall forward. During traction, the newborn pulls back against the examiner and usually shows flexion at the elbow, knee, and ankle (Fig. 1–3). The presence of more than minimal head lag and absence of any flexion of the arms in a term newborn during the traction response is abnormal (Fig. 1–4). Premature newborns of a gestational age of 33 weeks or older show greater head lag and less forceful flexion of the elbows, but the neck flexors consistently respond to the traction by lifting the head. Tests of traction in premature newborns less than 33 weeks' gestation are futile. A traction response is rare.

Next, test vertical suspension by placing both hands in the axillae, without grasping the thorax, and lifting straight up facing the examiner. The proximal muscles of the arms should be of sufficient strength to press down on the examiner's hands and allow the child to suspend vertically without falling through. While suspended, the child holds the head erect and in the midline for brief periods with flexion of the legs at the hips, knees, and ankles (Fig. 1–5). While in vertical suspension, the child's eyes frequently remain open; and lateral conjugate gaze is now testable, if not previously accomplished with the doll's eye maneuver. The examiner spins around while holding the child face to face at arm's length. This causes tonic lateral deviation in the direction opposite the movement of the head. Nystagmus does not occur.

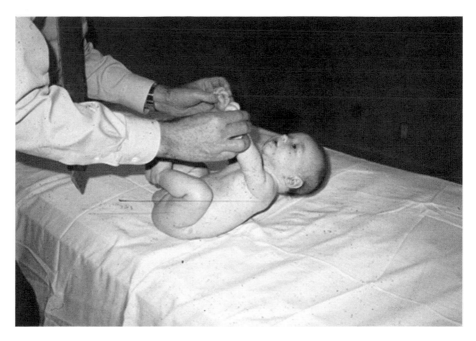

FIGURE 1–3 Normal traction response. The lift of the head is almost parallel to the lift of the body and there is flexion in all limb joints.

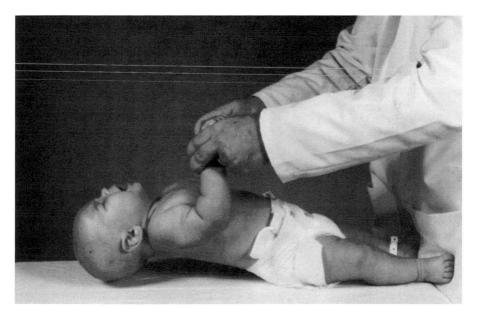

FIGURE 1–4 Abnormal traction response. The head falls backward as the body is pulled forward and there is no resistance to traction in the arms.

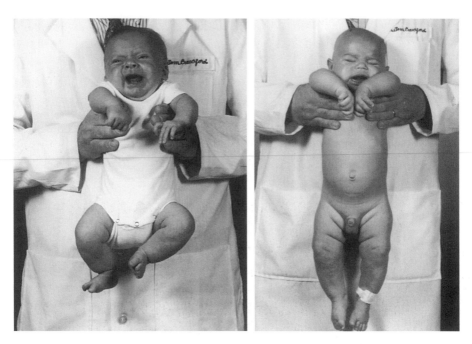

FIGURE 1–5   Normal vertical suspension. The head is in the midline and the limbs flex against gravity.

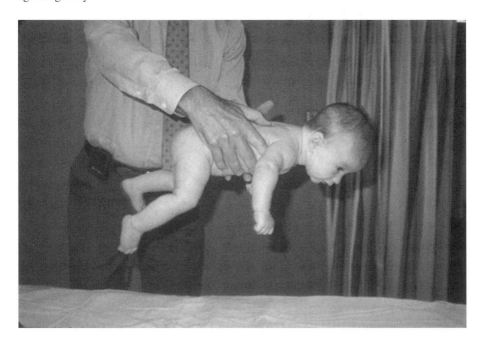

FIGURE 1–6   Normal horizontal suspension. The head rises intermittently and the head and limbs flex against gravity.

The examiner accomplishes horizontal suspension by placing the hands around the thorax without providing support for the head or legs (Fig. 1–6). The normal term newborn does not hang limply over the examiner's hand with the head and limbs dangling as in Figure 1–7. Instead, the back is held straight; flexion at the elbows, hips, knees, and ankles is observed; and at least brief attempts are made to keep the head erect (Fig. 1–6). The efforts become increasingly successful on each postpartum day. With the child in horizontal suspension, stroking the skin along the side of the vertebral column with a fingernail and observing an incurvature of the trunk with the concavity away from the painful stimulus tests *the Galant response.* This response may be useful as an aid in the localization of spinal cord lesions.

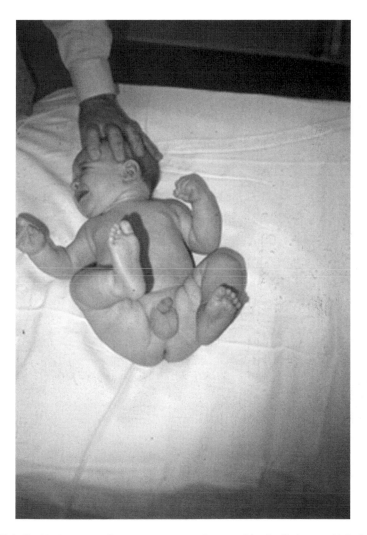

FIGURE 1–7 Tonic neck reflex. Extensor tone increased in the limbs to which the face is turned. Flexor tone increases in the contralateral limbs.

Integrated Reflexes

Among the transitory reflexes unique to the newborn infant, the Moro reflex, the tonic neck reflex, and the withdrawal reflex are routinely helpful in neurological assessment. Test these after completing the evaluation of tone.

The Moro Reflex

The Moro reflex is a startle reaction that allows observation of coordinated extension and flexion movements. The most effective and reproducible method for startling the newborn is the sensation of falling. The Moro reflex is, perhaps, the remnant of reflexes in newborn monkeys to maintain contact with a mother moving in the trees. With the child held in supine position, allow the head to fall a few centimeters, rapidly but gently, in the examiner's hands. The child's first response is a spreading movement in which the arms abduct and extend and the hands open. A clutching movement in which the arms adduct and flex over the body follows and the fists close. The spreading movement, but not the clutching, appears routinely in premature newborns at 28 weeks' gestation. Some extension of the legs is usually associated, but leg movements are not specifically part of the Moro reflex.

Complete absence of the spreading movement is always abnormal and most often observed in newborns with severe cerebral depression or disorders of the motor unit. Asymmetrical movements of the arms may indicate a palsy of the brachial plexus. An exaggerated Moro reflex, either because of a low threshold or because of excessive clutching, often occurs in newborns with moderate hypoxic-ischemic encephalopathy (see Ch. 4).

The Tonic Neck Reflex

After observing the Moro reflex, return the child to the supine position to test the tonic neck reflex. The tonic neck reflex is a primitive brainstem reflex that allows four-legged animals to pounce on prey. When a cat's head turns to the right in response to a moving target, the right forelimb extends and the left foreleg flexes. In humans, this brainstem 'pouncing' reflex is present at birth and then subdued by the maturation of the cerebral hemispheres.

With the head held in the midline, the limbs are in their resting flexion attitude. When the head turned to the right, extension tone increases in the right limbs and flexion tone increases in the left limbs. The only consistent visible evidence of these postural changes is extension of the arm. Extension of the leg is variable, and observable flexion in the contralateral limbs is rare. Nevertheless, the alteration in the distribution of tone is sufficient to increase the tendon reflexes on the side to which the face is turning and decrease the response on the opposite side. After observing the response to right head turning, rotate the head leftward to produce a reversal of posture (Fig. 1–8).

The tonic neck reflex is an important indicator of neurological abnormality if the responses are excessive and obligatory. In newborns with severe hemispheric dysfunction but an intact brainstem, turning of the head produces full

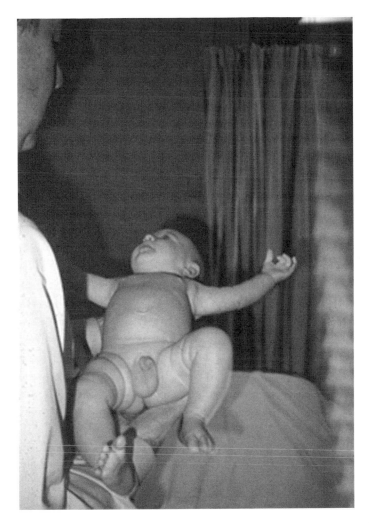

FIGURE 1–8 Moro reflex. The sensation of falling causes extension of the arms followed by flexion of the arms.

extension of both ipsilateral limbs and tight flexion on the contralateral side. These postures maintain for as long as the head remains rotated. This obligatory response is always abnormal; when unilateral it indicates brain damage in the hemisphere opposite to the extended limbs.

The Withdrawal Reflex

The withdrawal reflex is consistently present at 28 weeks' gestation and reflex integration is probably at a spinal level, since it is demonstrable in newborns with severe cerebral depression. Touching the sole of one foot with a pin provokes a flexion movement of the stimulated limb and extension of the contralateral limb. The contralateral extension is variable, and flexion of the opposite limb is a normal response. The absence of any flexion in the stimulated leg suggests a disorder of the motor unit.

Ophthalmoscopic Examination

Thorough inspection of the retina requires indirect ophthalmoscopic examination through a pharmacologically dilated pupil. The intention of this statement is not to discourage direct ophthalmoscopic examination, which readily provides information on the presence of two important abnormalities of the newborn: preretinal hemorrhages and chorioretinitis. The former is associated with intracranial hemorrhage and the latter suggests intracranial infection.

Direct ophthalmoscopy is most apt to be successful by placing the child in supine with the left side of the face resting on the surface and given a nipple to suck. In this position, most newborns open their eyes and keep them open for a sufficiently long period to permit examination of the right eye. Do not touch the child's face or eye, as this causes immediate lid closure. Instead, the examiner's free hand strokes the back of the head in order to maintain arousal. The examiner, standing rostral to the child's head, bends over and uses the right eye to look at the child's right eye. After completing the examination of the right eye, turn the child's head so that the right side of the face is down, and the process repeated with the left eye.

Head Circumference

Measure the head by determining its greatest anteroposterior circumference. Standards are available both for premature and for term newborns. The head circumference of newborns delivered from breech position averages 2 cm larger than that of newborns delivered from the vertex position. Excessive molding, cephalohematomas, and subgaleal infusions distort head circumference measurements.

Microcephaly at birth is evidence of antepartum disease. It is a major index of future neurological disability. An enlarged head may indicate hydrocephalus or intracranial bleeding and warrants further evaluation by CT or ultrasound.

BRAIN IMAGING

A joint committee of the American Academy of Neurology and the Child Neurology Society developed a practice parameter for Neuroimaging of newborns (Ment et al., 2002). They recommended routine screening cranial ultrasonography (US) for all newborns of 30 weeks' gestation between 7 and 14 days of age with repeat studies between 36 and 40 weeks' postmenstrual age. The purpose is to detect intraventricular hemorrhage, periventricular leukomalacia, and low-pressure ventriculomegaly. Such studies, in coordination with repeated clinical evaluations provide information concerning long-term neurodevelopmental outcome. Magnetic resonance imaging (MRI) in all very low birth weight preterm infants with abnormal cranial US results is not a recommendation. In the term infant, uncontrasted computerized tomography (CT) detects hemorrhagic lesions in encephalopathic term infants with a history of birth trauma, low hematocrit, or coagulopathy. MRI, between 2 and 8 days assess the location and extent of injury when CT findings are inconclusive. Basal ganglia and thalamic lesions detected by conventional MRI are associated with a poor neurodevelopmental outcome. Diffusion-weighted imaging may allow earlier detection of these cerebral injuries.

BRAIN DEATH

Published guidelines for the diagnosis of brain death often exclude newborns and even infants from consideration because published experience is lacking. Experience with the diagnosis of brain death in infants has been steadily increasing and newer guidelines do not differ substantially from those used in older children. The formal diagnosis of brain death in the newborn is a rare event; the basis for deciding to withdraw respiratory support is more often futility of care. A decision made jointly by the neonatologist and parents. Clinically suspect brain death in unarousable newborns, unable to sustain respiration, and without brainstem reflexes. Absence of cerebral blood flow using radionucleotide studies is confirmatory.

THE CONSULTATION NOTE

The birth of an imperfect child is often further burdened by feelings of guilt and anger. Often, nonphysicians scrutinize neurological consultation notes for purposes other than medical care. A factual presentation, written legibly and in precise language, best meets the needs of the child.

Clearly divide the history into the antepartum, intrapartum, and postpartum periods with the source of information stated. Detail the examination findings sufficiently to allow a comparison with subsequent observations. In writing the final formulation, it is helpful to summarize the specific historical events and points of examination that led to a diagnostic judgment. Table 1–2 summarizes the few critical features that cause neurological alarm. Recommendations should include, in addition to suggestions for treatment and laboratory studies, a comment indicating potential problems that will require continued vigilance. Avoid long-term prognosis in favor of repeat evaluations.

TABLE 1–2   Features associated with later neurological abnormality

Major features
1. Decreased states of consciousness
2. Increased intracranial pressure
3. Seizures
4. Hypotonia
5. Abnormal head size

Moderate features
1. Persistent deviation of head and/or eyes
2. Asymmetry of posture and/or movement

Minor features
1. Jitteriness
2. Poor feeding
3. Abnormal head shape

Most chronic handicapping conditions of the nervous system in children are present at the time of birth. The neurologist may have the unique opportunity to follow and study such children from birth onward. The information needed to provide early and effective plans of treatment often derive from the accurate recording of initial observations.

REFERENCES AND FURTHER READING

Amiel-Tison C, Maillard F, Lebrun F, et al. Neurological and physical maturation in normal growth and singletons from 37 to 41 weeks' gestation. Early Hum Dev 1999;54:145–156.

Fenichel GM. Neurological examination of the newborn. Brain Develop 1993;15:403–410.

Ment LR, Bada HS, Barnes P, et al. Practice parameter: Neuroimaging of the neonate. Report of the Quality Standards Subcommittee of the American Academy of Neurology and the Practice Committee of the Child Neurology Society. Neurology 2002;58:1726–1738.

Parker S, Zuckerman B, Bauchner H, et al. Jitteriness in full-term neonates: Prevalence and correlates. Pediatrics 1990;85:17–23.

2
Seizures

Gerald M. Fenichel

Seizures are an important feature of neurological disease in the newborn. The underlying cause of the seizures must be determined to initiate appropriate treatment. Further, uncontrolled seizures may contribute to further brain damage. Brain glucose decreases during prolonged seizures and excitatory amino acid release interferes with DNA synthesis. Therefore, seizures identified by electroencephalography (EEG) that occur without movement in newborns paralyzed with pancuronium are important to identify and treat.

SEIZURE PATTERNS

Table 2–1 lists clinical patterns associated with epileptiform discharges in newborns, while Table 2–2 lists movements often mistaken for seizures. The seizure classification is useful but does not do justice to the rich variety of patterns actually observed or take into account that 50% of prolonged epileptiform discharges on the electroencephalogram (EEG) are not associated with visible clinical changes. Generalized tonic clonic seizures do not occur. Many newborns suspected of having generalized tonic-clonic seizures are actually *jittery* (see Jitteriness, discussed later in this chapter). Newborns paralyzed with pancuronium to assist mechanical ventilation pose a special problem in seizure identification. In this circumstance, the presence of rhythmic increases in systolic arterial blood pressure, heart rate, and oxygenation should alert physicians to the possibility of seizures.

The definitive diagnosis of neonatal seizures often requires EEG monitoring. A split-screen 16-channel video-EEG is the ideal means for monitoring, but an ambulatory EEG capable of marking the time of events is serviceable. Epileptiform activity in the newborn is usually widespread and detectable even when the newborn is clinically asymptomatic.

Seizures in newborns, especially those who are premature, are poorly organized and difficult to distinguish from normal activity. Newborns with

TABLE 2–1   Seizure patterns in newborns

Apnea with tonic stiffening of body
Focal clonic movements of one limb or both limbs on one side
Multifocal clonic limb movements
Myoclonic jerking
Paroxysmal laughing
Tonic deviation of the eyes upward or to one side
Tonic stiffening of the body

From Fenichel (2005) Clinical Pediatric Neurology: A Signs and Symptoms Approach, 5th edn. Elsevier Saunders.

hydranencephaly or atelencephaly are capable of generating the full variety of neonatal seizure patterns. This supports the notion that seizures may arise from the brainstem as well as the hemispheres and remain confined there by the absence of myelinated pathways for cortical propagation. For the same reason, seizures originating in one hemisphere are unlikely to spread beyond the contiguous cortex or to produce secondary bilateral synchrony.

Five clinical seizure patterns occur in newborns: subtle, multifocal clonic, focal clonic, tonic, and myoclonic. Tonic-clonic seizures do not occur. EEG evidence of epileptiform activity, even electrical status epilepticus, may also occur in nonparalyzed newborns, especially prematures, without any outward sign of seizures. Such newborns usually are flaccid and unresponsive during the time when the EEG records epileptiform activity.

Subtle Seizures

The term *subtle seizures* encompasses several patterns of seizures in which tonic and clonic movements of the limbs are lacking (Table 2–3). Instead, behavioral changes or movements occur that are indistinguishable from normal movements by even an experienced examiner. The results of EEG monitoring studies have confirmed the difficulty of clinical observation and underlined the need for concomitant EEG for certainty in diagnosis. Exceptions are tonic deviation of the eyes in term newborns and ocular fixation with sustained eye opening in prematures. These are usually seizure manifestations (Volpe, 2001). Epileptiform

TABLE 2–2   Movements that resemble neonatal seizures

Benign nocturnal myoclonus
Jitteriness
Nonconvulsive apnea
Normal movement
Opisthotonos
Pathological myoclonus

From Fenichel. (2005) Clinical Pediatric Neurology: A Signs and Symptoms Approach, 5th edn. Elsevier Saunders.

TABLE 2–3   Subtle seizure patterns in newborns

Apnea
Tonic deviation of the eyes
Repetitive fluttering of eyelids
Drooling, sucking, chewing
Swimming movements of the arms
Pedaling movements of the legs
Paroxysmal laughing

discharges do not accompany the tonic extensor posturing of newborns with severe intraventricular hemorrhage and anticonvulsant therapy does not change the posturing (Sher, 1997).

Apnea is rarely a seizure manifestation unless associated with tonic deviation of the eyes. Bradycardia may not be associated even when apnea is prolonged. With continuous respiratory monitoring, apneic spells are detectable at some time in almost all prematures and in many normal term newborns. The highest incidence is during active sleep. When prematures reach 40 weeks conceptional age, they continue to show a higher incidence of apneic spells than do 40 week term newborns.

Multifocal Clonic Seizures

Multifocal clonic seizures are migratory. Clonic movements shift from one limb to another without following any pattern of gyral or callosal spread. In some seizures, the clonic movements migrate rapidly from limb to limb and from side to side. In others, prolonged focal clonic movements occur in one limb before commencing in another. EEG monitoring shows shifting sites of epileptiform activity associated with the shifting sites of clinical seizures. The usual cause of this seizure pattern is a generalized cerebral disturbance such as hypoxic-ischemic encephalopathy.

Focal Clonic Seizures

The cause of clonic seizures that remain localized to one limb or one side is invariably a cerebrovascular event, either an infarction or an intracerebral hemorrhage. Slow clonic movements (1 to 3 jerks/second) usually begin in a single limb or on one side of the face and may spread to involve other body parts on the same side without loss of consciousness. Faster clonic movements (3 to 4 jerks/second), confined to circumscribed muscle groups, occur in the fingers, hands, or feet. Each jerk is consistently associated with focal rhythmic sharp-wave EEG discharges in the contralateral central region. When the jerking of one limb spreads to involve the other limb on the same side, the EEG discharge spreads to involve much of the contralateral hemisphere.

Tonic Seizures

Generalized, tonic stiffening of the body, characterized by hyperextension of the limbs, is relatively common in newborns. Such episodes are rarely seizures. In contrast, generalized stiffening of the body associated with tonic deviation of the eyes, and asymmetrical posturing of the limbs on one side are closely associated with concomitant EEG epileptiform activity. Most tonic posturing in stressed newborns probably represents a transitory disinhibition of normal tonic brainstem facilitation due to forebrain dysfunction. Prolonged disinhibition produces decerebrate rigidity. Decerebrate posturing and opisthotonos are different from other causes of tonic stiffening and have different diagnostic and therapeutic implications.

Myoclonic Seizures

Synchronized jerking movements of either the arms or legs, or both, are uncommon in newborns as a seizure manifestation. When present, they have an inconsistent relationship to EEG seizure discharges. Myoclonic jerks in newborns with decreased states of consciousness due to inborn errors of metabolism are often seizure manifestations. Myoclonic seizures may evolve into infantile spasms and have a poor prognosis. EEG distinguishes seizures from *benign neonatal sleep myoclonus*. Repeated flexion movements of the fingers, wrist, and elbows during sleep characterize benign sleep myoclonus. The EEG is normal, the child appears normal on examination, and the movements stop upon awakening. Jitteriness, a hyperirritable state seen in some stressed newborns, is frequently confused with myoclonic seizures. Chapter 1 summarizes the important points of distinction.

SEIZURE-LIKE EVENTS

Apnea

- **Clinical features.** An irregular respiratory pattern with intermittent pauses of 3 to 6 seconds, often followed by 10 to 15 seconds of hyperpnea, is a common occurrence in premature infants. The pauses are not associated with significant alterations in heart rate, blood pressure, body temperature, or skin color. Immaturity of the brainstem respiratory centers causes this respiratory pattern, termed *periodic breathing*. The incidence of periodic breathing correlates directly with the degree of prematurity. Apneic spells are more common during active than during quiet sleep.

    Apneic spells of 10 to 15 seconds are detectable at some time in almost all premature and some full-term newborns. Apneic spells of 10 to 20 seconds are usually associated with a 20% reduction in heart rate. Longer episodes of apnea are almost invariably associated with a 40% or greater reduction in heart rate. The frequency of these apneic spells correlates with brainstem myelination. Even at 40 weeks conceptional age, premature newborns continue to have a higher incidence of apnea than do full-term newborns. The incidence of apnea sharply decreases in all infants at 52 weeks conceptional age.

- **Diagnosis.** Apneic spells in an otherwise normal-appearing newborn is a sign of brainstem immaturity and not a pathological condition. The sudden onset of apnea and states of decreased consciousness, especially in premature newborns, suggests an intracranial hemorrhage with brainstem compression. Immediate ultrasound examination is in order.

  Apneic spells are almost never a seizure manifestation unless they are associated with tonic deviation of the eyes, tonic stiffening of the body, or characteristic limb movements. *However, prolonged apnea without bradycardia, and especially with tachycardia, is a seizure until proven otherwise.*
- **Management.** Short episodes of apnea do not require intervention.

Benign Nocturnal Myoclonus

- **Clinical features.** Sudden jerking movements of the limbs during sleep occur in normal people of all ages (see Ch. 14). They appear primarily during the early stages of sleep as repeated flexion movements of the fingers, wrists, and elbows. The jerks do not localize consistently, stop with gentle restraint, and end abruptly with arousal. When prolonged, the usual misdiagnosis is focal clonic or myoclonic seizures.
- **Diagnosis.** The distinction between nocturnal myoclonus and seizures or jitteriness is that it occurs solely during sleep, is not activated by a stimulus, and the EEG is normal.
- **Management.** Treatment is not required. Anticonvulsant drugs may increase the frequency of benign nocturnal myoclonus by causing sedation.

Jitteriness

- **Clinical features.** Jitteriness or tremulousness is an excessive response to stimulation. Touch, noise, or motion provokes a low frequency, high-amplitude shaking of the limbs and jaw. Jitteriness is commonly associated with a low threshold for the Moro reflex, but it can occur in the absence of any apparent stimulation and be confused with myoclonic seizures.
- **Diagnosis.** Jitteriness usually occurs in newborns with perinatal asphyxia that may have seizures as well. EEG monitoring, the absence of eye movements or alteration in respiratory pattern, and the presence of stimulus activation distinguishes jitteriness from seizures. Newborns of addicted mothers and newborns with metabolic disorders are also jittery.
- **Management.** Reduced stimulation decreases jitteriness. However, newborns of addicted mothers require sedation to facilitate feeding and to decrease energy expenditure.

DIFFERENTIAL DIAGNOSIS

Virtually any stress to the newborn nervous system, whether primary to the brain or secondary to a systemic disorder, can cause a seizure. In assessing a newborn with seizures, it is important to consider multiple causes. One example of cumulative risk is the newborn of a diabetic mother in whom dysmaturity, hypoglycemia, and sepsis may coexist. A second example is prematurity and its association with hypoglycemia, hypocalcemia, sepsis, anoxia, and intraventricular hemorrhage. The importance of multiple risk factors in the pathogenesis of neonatal seizures is to stress the need for a therapeutic plan that treats all causes.

Table 2–4 classifies neonatal seizures by peak time of onset. This is the most practical approach to differential diagnosis. An additional approach is to consider the child's condition prior to the onset of seizures. In the following situations, newborns are generally comatose, or at least quite lethargic, before they experience seizures: (a) hypoxic-ischemic encephalopathy; (b) traumatic intracerebral hemorrhage; (c) periventricular-intraventricular hemorrhage of prematurity; and (d) inborn errors of metabolism. Newborns with seizures caused by cerebral dysgenesis often have dysmorphic features or malformations of other

TABLE 2–4   Differential diagnosis of neonatal seizures by peak time of onset

24 hours
Bacterial meningitis and sepsis
Direct drug effect
Hypoxic-ischemic encephalopathy
Intrauterine infection
Intraventricular hemorrhage at term
Laceration of tentorium or falx
Pyridoxine dependency
Subarachnoid hemorrhage

24 to 72 hours
Bacterial meningitis and sepsis
Cerebral contusion with subdural hemorrhage
Cerebral dysgenesis
Cerebral infarction
Drug withdrawal
Glycine encephalopathy
Glycogen synthase deficiency
Hypoparathyroidism–hypocalcemia
Idiopathic cerebral venous thrombosis
Incontinentia pigmenti
Intracerebral hemorrhage
Intraventricular hemorrhage in premature newborns
Pyridoxine dependency
Subarachnoid hemorrhage
Tuberous sclerosis
Urea cycle disturbances

TABLE 2–4   Differential diagnosis of neonatal seizures by peak time of onset—Cont'd

72 hours to 1 week
Familial neonatal seizures
Cerebral dysgenesis
Cerebral infarction
Hypoparathyroidism
Idiopathic cerebral venous thrombosis
Intracerebral hemorrhage
Kernicterus
Methylmalonic acidemia
Nutritional hypocalcemia
Propionic acidemia
Tuberous sclerosis
Urea cycle disturbances

1 to 4 weeks
Adrenoleukodystrophy, neonatal
Cerebral dysgenesis
Fructose dysmetabolism
Gaucher disease type 2
GM_1 gangliosidosis type 1
Herpes simplex encephalitis
Idiopathic cerebral venous thrombosis
Ketotic hyperglycinemias
Maple syrup urine disease, neonatal
Tuberous sclerosis
Urea cycle disturbances

From Fenichel. (2005) Clinical Pediatric Neurology: A Signs and Symptoms Approach, 5th edn. Elsevier Saunders.

organs, and those with intrauterine infections have evidence of systemic involvement; that is growth retardation, rash, jaundice, hepatosplenomegaly, and chorioretinitis. When a seizure occurs in a newborn that had previously appeared relatively well, one should consider sepsis, subarachnoid hemorrhage, cerebral infarction, intracerebral hemorrhage, hypocalcemia, and benign familial neonatal seizures.

Table 2–5 lists those conditions that are not ordinarily associated with neonatal seizures. Chromosomal aberrations are sometimes associated with such severe neonatal hypotonia that respiration is impaired, and the consequent asphyxia causes seizures.

TABLE 2–5   Disorders not usually associated with neonatal seizures

Chromosomal aberrations
Homocystinuria and phenylketonuria
Inborn errors of lipid metabolism
Inborn errors of metal metabolism
Inborn errors of mucopolysaccharide metabolism
Inborn errors resulting in glycogen storage
Maternal use of alcohol, anticonvulsants, marijuana, and sedatives

Bilirubin Encephalopathy

Unconjugated bilirubin is bound to albumin in the blood. *Kernicterus*, a yellow discoloration of the brain that is especially severe in the basal ganglia and hippocampus, occurs when the serum unbound or free fraction becomes excessive. An excessive level of the free fraction in an otherwise healthy newborn is approximately 20 mg/dL (340 μmol/L). Kernicterus was an important complication of hemolytic disease from maternal-fetal blood group incompatibility, but this condition is now uncommon. The management of other causes of hyperbilirubinemia in full-term newborns is not difficult. Critically ill premature infants with respiratory distress syndrome, acidosis, and sepsis are the group at greatest risk. In such newborns, an unbound serum concentration of 10 mg/dL (170 μmol/L) may be sufficient to cause bilirubin encephalopathy, and even the albumin-bound fraction may pass the blood–brain barrier.

Clinical Features   Three distinct clinical phases of bilirubin encephalopathy occur in full-term newborns with untreated hemolytic disease. Hypotonia, lethargy, and a poor sucking reflex occur within 24 hours of delivery. Bilirubin staining of the brain is already evident in newborns dying during this first clinical phase. On the second or third day, the newborn becomes febrile and shows increasing tone and opisthotonic posturing. Seizures are not a constant feature but may occur at this time. Characteristic of the third phase is apparent improvement with normalization of tone. This may cause second thoughts about the accuracy of the diagnosis, but the improvement is short-lived. Evidence of neurological dysfunction begins to appear toward the end of the second month, and the symptoms become progressively worse throughout infancy.

In premature newborns, the clinical features are subtle and may lack the phases of increased tone and opisthotonos.

The typical clinical syndrome after the first year includes extrapyramidal dysfunction, usually athetosis, which occurs in virtually every case (see Ch. 14); disturbances of vertical gaze, upward more often than downward, in 90%; high-frequency hearing loss in 60%; and mental retardation in 25%.

Diagnosis   In newborns with hemolytic disease, the basis for a presumed clinical diagnosis is a significant hyperbilirubinemia and a compatible evolution of symptoms. However, the diagnosis is difficult to establish in critically ill premature newborns, in which the cause of brain damage is more often asphyxia than kernicterus.

The brainstem auditory evoked response (BAER) may be useful in assessing the severity of bilirubin encephalopathy and its response to treatment. The auditory nerve and pathways are especially susceptible to bilirubin encephalopathy. The generators of wave I and wave V of the BAER are the auditory nerve and the inferior colliculus, respectively. The latency of both waves increases in proportion to the concentration of free albumin and decreases after exchange transfusion.

Management   Maintaining serum bilirubin concentrations below the toxic range, either by phototherapy or exchange transfusion, prevents kernicterus.

Once kernicterus has occurred, further damage can be limited, but not reversed, by lowering serum bilirubin concentrations.

Drugs

Fetal exposure to drugs is through maternal use. Table 2–6 summarizes major adverse effects of neuroactive drugs administered during pregnancy. Marihuana, alcohol, narcotic-analgesics, and other hypnotic sedatives are the drugs most commonly used habitually, either alone or in combination, during pregnancy. Marihuana and alcohol do not cause drug dependence in the fetus and therefore are not associated with withdrawal symptoms in the newborn. Marijuana use during pregnancy does not affect the fetus adversely. Although maternal

TABLE 2–6   Adverse effects of neuroactive drugs administered during pregnancy

Neuroactive drugs	*Passive addiction*	*Known teratogenic*	*Neonatal seizures*	*Intrauterine growth retardation*	*Coagulation disorders (neonatal intracranial hemorrhage)*
Alcohol	+	+	+	+	
Heroin/methadone	+		+ (methadone)	+	
Cocaine	+	+	?	+	
Benzodiazepines	+				
Tricyclic antidepressants	+		+		
Hydroxyzine (Atarax)	+				
Ethchlorvynol (Placidyl)	+				
Propoxyphene (Darvon)	+		+		
Pentazocine (Talwin)	+				
'Ts and blues' (pentazocine, tripelennamine)	+		+		
Codeine	+				
Hydantoins		+			+
Barbiturates	+	+	+ (short-acting)		+
Primidone	+	+			+
Valproate		+		±	
Oxazolidine derivatives (trimethadione)		+		+	

+ = present; ± = possibly present.

From Hill. Neurology in Clinical Practice, 4th edn. Elsevier.

alcoholism produces a distinctive array of multisystem malformations (*the fetal alcohol syndrome*), the syndrome is not associated with neonatal seizures. Other substances of abuse come into and out of favor and most produce some adverse reaction to the fetus. Other prenatal maternal behaviors such as poor nutrition, poor prenatal care, and maternal infection further magnify the poor outcome for the fetus.

Maternal use of cocaine during pregnancy is frequently associated with small birth weight, premature delivery, abruptio placenta, and fetal vascular changes that may cause stroke or limb abnormalities. Newborns exposed to cocaine in utero or postpartum through the breast milk may show features of cocaine intoxication: tachycardia, tachypnea, hypertension, irritability, and tremulousness. Phenobarbital provides sedation until the symptoms disappear during the second or third week.

Narcotic-Analgesic Withdrawal

The prototype for neonatal narcotic-analgesic withdrawal is heroin, but an identical syndrome occurs with legally prescribed narcotics used as a cough suppressant and non-narcotic analgesics such as propoxyphene given to the mother just before delivery. The onset of symptoms depends to some extent on the weight of the child (small newborns become symptomatic sooner than larger newborns), and the amount of time between the mother's last dose and the time of delivery. Seventy percent begin withdrawal during the first 24 hours and almost all the remainder within 48 hours. The withdrawal begins with a vigorous course tremor that can shake an entire limb and is present only in the waking state. The child becomes extremely irritable, has a shrill high-pitched cry, and is in constant motion. Despite ravenous hunger, feeding is difficult and followed by vomiting. Diarrhea and other symptoms of autonomic instability are common. Rigidity of the limbs occurs in which there is resistance to either flexion or extension. Myoclonic jerking occurs in 10 to 25% of newborns of addicted mothers, but these movements are more likely jitteriness than seizures. Definite seizures occur in less than 2% of newborns undergoing heroin withdrawal but may occur in 8% undergoing methadone withdrawal.

If left untreated, the symptoms remit spontaneously within 3 to 5 days, but the mortality is appreciable. Phenobarbital 8 mg/kg/day and chlorpromazine 3 mg/kg/day in divided doses are equally effective in alleviating most of the symptoms and in reducing mortality. Phenobarbital is useful in the treatment of neonatal methadone withdrawal as well. The quantities of morphine, opium, meperidine, and methadone secreted in breast milk are insufficient to cause addiction or to relieve withdrawal symptoms in the newborn.

Hypnotic-Sedative Withdrawal

Dependence on hypnotic-sedatives, such as phenobarbital, is common in children of epileptic mothers. These newborns are not small for gestational age (SGA) and do not have an increased incidence of perinatal complications.

Maternal phenobarbital doses of 60 to 120 mg/day during the last trimester are sufficient to produce fetal drug dependence. The withdrawal symptoms begin 3 to 7 days after delivery and may last for up to 6 months. The syndrome is not unlike that encountered in older children given phenobarbital: hyperexcitability, tremor, restlessness, and difficulty sleeping. Seizures are uncommon, perhaps because the very long half-life of phenobarbital serves as a protection against abrupt withdrawal.

Metabolic Disturbances

Several inborn errors of metabolism may cause neonatal seizures. Chapter 7 details these disorders, but Table 2–7 summarizes the screening tests that suggest a metabolic disorder causing seizures in newborns. As a general rule, newborns with hyperammonemia appear systemically sick before the onset of seizures.

TABLE 2–7 **Screening for inborn errors of metabolism that cause neonatal seizures**

Blood glucose low
Fructose 1,6,-diphosphatase deficiency
Glycogen storage disease, type 1
Maple syrup urine disease

Blood calcium low
Hypoparathyroidism
Maternal hyperparathyroidism

Blood ammonia high
Argininosuccinic acidemia
Carbamylphosphate synthetase deficiency
Citrullinemia
Methylmalonic acidemia (may be normal)
Multiple carboxylase deficiency
Ornithine transcarbamylase deficiency
Propionic acidemia (may be normal)

Blood lactate high
Fructose 1,6,-diphosphatase deficiency
Glycogen storage disease, type 1
Mitochondrial disorders
Multiple carboxylase deficiency

Metabolic acidosis
Fructose 1,6,-diphosphatase deficiency
Glycogen storage disease, type 1
Maple syrup urine disease
Methylmalonic acidemia
Multiple carboxylase deficiency
Propionic acidemia

From Fenichel. (2005) Clinical Pediatric Neurology: A Signs and Symptoms Approach, 5th edn. Elsevier Saunders.

Hypoglycemia

The traditional definition of neonatal hypoglycemia is a whole blood glucose level of less than 20 mg/dL in premature newborns and low-birth weight newborns, less than 30 mg/dL in term newborns during the first 72 hours, and less than 40 mg/dL in any newborn after 72 hours. A transitory asymptomatic hypoglycemia occurs in approximately 10% of all newborns during the first 6 hours and before the first feeding. The hypoglycemia responds well to oral feeding and is not associated with neurological handicaps later in life.

By contrast, *symptomatic hypoglycemia* is secondary to a specific stress or pathological state (Table 2–8). Clinical manifestations of cerebral dysfunction during hypoglycemia indicate a significant risk of permanent brain damage. The onset and progression of symptoms vary with the underlying process but are always manifest within the first 72 hours. The syndrome includes any combination of the following: apnea, cyanosis, tachypnea, jitteriness, a high-pitched cry, difficulty feeding, vomiting, apathy, hypotonia, seizures, and coma.

TABLE 2–8   Causes of neonatal hypoglycemia

Primary transitional hypoglycemia
Complicated labor and delivery
Intrauterine malnutrition
Maternal diabetes
Prematurity

Secondary transitional hypoglycemia
Asphyxia
Central nervous system disorders
Cold injuries
Sepsis

Persistent hypoglycemia
Aminoacidurias
Maple syrup urine disease
Methylmalonic acidemia
Propionic acidemia
Tyrosinosis
Congenital hypopituitarism
Defects in carbohydrate metabolism
Fructose 1,6-diphosphatase deficiency
Fructose + intolerance
Galactosemia
Glycogen storage disease, type 1
Glycogen synthase deficiency
Hyperinsulinism
Organic acidurias
Glutaric aciduria type 2
3-Methyl glutaryl-CoA lyase deficiency

From Fenichel. (2005) Clinical Pediatric Neurology: A Signs and Symptoms Approach, 5th edn. Elsevier Saunders.

Hypoglycemia is rarely the only etiological factor in newborns with seizures. The prognosis in newborns with hypoglycemia and seizures usually depends upon the underlying causes. Prolonged and severe episodes of hypoglycemia have a deleterious effect on the nervous system and require treatment along with the underlying causes. In urgent situations characterized by seizures, apnea, and hypotension, 0.5 to 1.0 g/kg of glucose is administered intravenously (IV) as 2 to 4 mL/kg of a 25% solution. Glucose infusions of 8 mg/kg/min follow as needed.

A persistent but later-onset hypoglycemia of sufficient severity to cause seizures occurs in fructose intolerance, fructose-1,6-diphosphatase deficiency, and glycogen synthase deficiency. Chapter 7 details these disorders. Maple syrup urine disease, propionic acidemia, and methymalonic acidemia are also associated with hypoglycemia and seizures, but biochemical derangements other than hypoglycemia are present that may contribute to the seizure tendency.

Hypocalcemia

The definition of hypocalcemia is a blood calcium concentration less than 7 mg/dL (1.75 mmol/L). The onset of hypocalcemia in the first 72 hours after delivery is associated with low birth weight, asphyxia, maternal diabetes, transitory neonatal hypoparathyroidism, maternal hyperparathyroidism, and the DiGeorge syndrome. Later-onset hypocalcemia occurs in children fed evaporated cow's milk and other improper formulas, in maternal hyperparathyroidism, and in the DiGeorge syndrome.

Hypoparathyroidism in the newborn may result from maternal hyperparathyroidism or may be a transitory phenomenon of unknown cause. Hypocalcemia occurs in less than 10% of stressed newborns and enhances their vulnerability to seizures, but it is rarely the primary cause.

DiGeorge syndrome (22q11.1 microdeletion syndrome) The DiGeorge syndrome is associated with microdeletions of chromosome 22q11.2 (McDonald-McGinn et al., 2004). Disturbance of cervical neural crest migration into the derivatives of the pharyngeal arches and pouches explains the phenotype. Organs derived from the third and fourth pharyngeal pouches (thymus, parathyroid gland, and great vessels) are hypoplastic.

- **Clinical features.** The 22q11.2 *deletion* syndrome encompasses two *phenotypes*: DiGeorge syndrome (DGS) and *velocardiofacial syndrome* (VCFS) (Shprintzen syndrome). The acronym CATCH is used to describe the phenotype of cardiac abnormality, T-cell deficit, clefting (multiple minor facial anomalies), and hypocalcemia. The identification of most children with DGS is in the neonatal period with a major *congenital* heart defect, hypocalcemia, and immunodeficiency. Diagnosis of children with VCFS comes later because of cleft palate or craniofacial deformities.
- The initial symptoms of DGS may be due to congenital heart disease, hypocalcemia, or both. Jitteriness and tetany usually begin in the first 48 hours after delivery. The peak onset of seizures is on the third day but a 2-week

delay may occur. Many affected newborns die of cardiac causes during the first month; survivors fail to thrive and have frequent infections because of the failure of cell-mediated immunity.

- **Diagnosis.** Newborns with DGS come to medical attention because of seizures and heart disease. Seizures or a prolonged Q-T interval brings attention to hypocalcemia. Molecular genetic testing confirms the diagnosis.
- **Management.** Management requires a multispecialty team including cardiology, immunology, medical genetics, and neurology. Plastic surgery, dentistry, and child development contribute later on. Hypocalcemia generally responds to parathyroid hormone or to oral calcium and vitamin D.

A prolonged Q-T interval on the electrocardiogram (ECG) suggests hypocalcemia in newborns coming to attention because of heart disease. Conversely, all newborns with symptoms of hypocalcemia require an examination for cardiac defects. Hypocalcemia generally responds to parathyroid hormone or to oral calcium and vitamin D.

Hypomagnesemia

Primary hypomagnesemia is a rare autosomal recessive genetic disease due to magnesium malabsorption. Seizures are the primary manifestation. Delays of seizure onset may be as long as three months. Hypocalcemia is present as well and treatment may be misdirected. The seizures respond only to parenteral administration of magnesium. Early treatment results in normal development but delay in treatment causes permanent neurological impairment.

Other Genetic Defects

Inborn errors of metabolism that lead to the abnormal storage of carbohydrates, mucopolysaccharides, lipids, and metals can cause systemic disturbances and hypotonia during the neonatal period but are not associated with early seizures. Two exceptions are GalNAc transferase deficiency (G_{m3} gangliosidosis) and infantile gangliosidosis Type I. Chapter 7 details these rare disorders of ganglioside metabolism.

Benign Familial Neonatal Seizures

In some families, several members have seizures in the first weeks of life but do not have epilepsy or other neurological abnormalities later on. Transmission of the trait is autosomal dominant and abnormal gene loci map to chromosomes 20q and 8q. The mutations are in the voltage gated potassium genes (Lerche et al., 2001).

- **Clinical features.** Brief multifocal clonic seizures develop during the first week, sometimes associated with apnea. Delay of onset may be as long as 4 weeks. With or without treatment, the seizures usually stop spontaneously within 6 weeks. Febrile seizures occur in up to one third of affected

children; some have febrile seizures without first having neonatal seizures. Epilepsy develops later in life in 10% to 15% of affected newborns.
- **Diagnosis.** Suspect the syndrome when seizures develop without apparent cause in a healthy newborn. Laboratory tests, including the interictal EEG, are normal. During a seizure, the initial apnea and tonic activity are associated with flattening of the EEG; generalized spike-wave discharges occur during the clonic activity. A family history of neonatal seizures is critical to diagnosis but may await discovery until interviewing the grandparents; parents are frequently unaware that they had neonatal seizures.
- **Management.** Phenobarbital usually stops seizures. After 4 weeks of complete seizure control, taper and discontinue the drug. Initiate a longer trial if seizures recur.

Benign Familial Neonatal–Infantile Seizures

The onset of a second benign genetic epilepsy syndrome is anytime from three days to six months. The genetic defect is missense mutations in the sodium channel (Berkovic et al., 2004). Febrile seizures are uncommon. The seizures are partial in onset and then become generalized. Seizures stop by age 12 months.

Incontinentia Pigmenti

Incontinentia pigmenti is a rare neurocutaneous syndrome involving the skin, teeth, eyes, and central nervous system. Genetic transmission is X-linked (Xq28) with lethality in the hemizygous male (Scheuerle, 2003).

- **Clinical features.** The female-to-male ratio is 20:1. An erythematous and vesicular rash resembling epidermolysis bullosa is present on the flexor surfaces of the limbs and lateral aspect of the trunk at birth or soon thereafter. The rash persists for the first few months and a verrucous eruption that lasts for weeks or months replaces the original rash. Between 6 and 12 months of age, deposits of pigment appear in the previous area of rash in bizarre polymorphic arrangements. The pigmentation later regresses and leaves a linear hypopigmentation. Alopecia, hypodontia, abnormal tooth shape, and dystrophic nails may be associated. Some have retinal vascular abnormalities that predispose to retinal detachment in early childhood.
  Neurological disturbances occur in fewer than half of the cases. In newborns, the prominent feature is the onset of seizures on the second or third day, often confined to one side of the body. Residual neurological handicaps may include mental retardation, epilepsy, hemiparesis, and hydrocephalus.
- **Diagnosis.** The clinical findings and biopsy of the skin rash are diagnostic. *Molecular genetic testing* of the IKBKG *gene* reveals mutations in about 80% of *probands.*
- **Management.** Neonatal seizures caused by incontinentia pigmenti usually respond to standard anticonvulsant drugs. The blistering rash requires topical medication and oatmeal baths. Regular ophthalmological examinations manage retinal detachment.

Pyridoxine Dependency

Pyridoxine dependency is a rare disorder transmitted as an autosomal recessive trait (Gospe, 2002). The genetic locus is unknown but the presumed cause is impaired glutamic decarboxylase activity.

- **Clinical features.** Newborns experience seizures soon after birth. The seizures are usually multifocal clonic at onset and progress rapidly to status epilepticus. Although presentations consisting of prolonged seizures and recurrent episodes of status epilepticus are typical, recurrent self-limited events including partial seizures, generalized seizures, atonic seizures, myoclonic events, and infantile spasms also occur. The seizures only respond to pyridoxine. A seizure-free interval up to three weeks may occur after pyridoxine discontinuation. Intellectual disability is common.

  An atypical form includes seizure-onset up to two years of age. The seizures initially respond to anticonvulsants and then become intractable.
- **Diagnosis.** In most cases, the diagnosis is suspected because an affected older sibling. In the absence of a family history, suspect the diagnosis in newborns with continuous seizures. Characteristic of the infantile-onset variety is intermittent myoclonic seizures, focal clonic seizures, or generalized tonic-clonic seizures. The EEG is continuously abnormal because of generalized or multifocal spike discharges. An intravenous injection of pyridoxine, 100 mg, stops the clinical seizure activity and often converts the EEG to normal in less than 10 minutes. However, sometimes 500 mg is required.
- **Management.** A lifelong dietary supplement of pyridoxine, which varies from 10 to 50 mg/kg/day, prevents further seizures. Subsequent psychomotor development is best with early treatment, but this does not ensure a normal outcome. The dose needed to prevent mental retardation may be higher than that needed to stop seizures.

TREATMENT

Neonatal seizures require urgent treatment. Once adequate ventilation and perfusion are established, the blood glucose concentration is measured. If the glucose concentration is low, administer 10% dextrose in a dose of 2 mL/kg. In the absence of hypoglycemia, initiate immediate treatment with anticonvulsant medications. Studies to determine other underlying causes proceed concurrently, and specific treatment initiated when possible.

Phenobarbital alone controls seizures in most newborns at loading dosages up to 40 mg/kg. A fosphenytoin infusion, 20 mg/kg, is the next drug used if seizures continue. Most seizures usually respond to intravenous loading doses of phenobarbital and fosphenytoin. When these drugs fail, it is unlikely that benzodiazepines will prove effective and barbiturate coma is preferable.

Phenobarbital may suppress seizures caused by hypocalcemia, and a favorable response does not exclude that diagnosis. Approximately 50% of newborns with hypocalcemia also have hypomagnesemia, which requires specific treatment.

Duration of Treatment

The optimal duration of maintenance therapy for neonatal seizures is unknown. The duration of maintenance treatment for neonatal seizures depends on the risk of recurrence and the underlying cause. The treatment of seizures secondary to an acute self-limited encephalopathy, such as caused by asphyxia, does not ordinarily require prolonged maintenance therapy. In most newborns, seizures cease spontaneously within 7 to 14 days as the acute encephalopathy subsides. The incidence of later epilepsy among infants who have had neonatal seizures secondary to perinatal asphyxia or intracranial injury is about 30%. In contrast to acute self-limited encephalopathies, the incidence of later epilepsy in newborns with seizures from cerebral dysgenesis is 80%. Such seizures usually continue from the newborn period directly into infancy and childhood requiring continuous anticonvulsant therapy.

Discontinue phenytoin when intravenous therapy stops. Maintenance of adequate serum levels oral phenytoin is not possible in the newborn. If seizures have stopped and the neurological examination and EEG are normal, discontinue phenobarbital before hospital discharge. When continuing phenobarbital after hospital discharge, consider discontinuation as early as 1 month later based on the neurological status and EEG. Discontinue phenobarbital in an infant whose examination is not normal if the EEG does not show epileptiform activity.

REFERENCES AND FURTHER READING

Berkovic S, Heron SE, Giordano L, et al. Benign familial neonatal-infantile seizures: Characterization of a new sodium channelopathy. Ann Neurol 2004;55:550–557.

Gospe SM. Pyridoxine-dependent seizures: findings from recent studies pose new questions. Pediatr Neurol 2002;26:181–185.

Lerche H, Jukott-Ratt K and Lehmann-Horn F. Ions channels and epilepsy. Am J Med Genet 2001;106:146–159.

McDonald-McGinn DM, Emanuel MS and Zackai EH. 22q11.2 Deletion Syndrome (23 July 2004). In: GeneClinics: Medical Genetics Knowledge Base. [database online] University of Washington, Seattle. Available at http://www.geneclinics.org

Roland EH and Hill A. Intraventricular hemorrhage and posthemorrhagic hydrocephalus. Clin Perinatol 1997;24:589–605.

Roland EH, Poskitt K, Rodriguez E, et al. Perinatal hypoxic-ischemic thalamic injury: Clinical features and neuroimaging. Ann Neurol 1998;44:161–166.

Scheuerle AE. Incontinentia pigmenti. (27 March 2003) In: GeneClinics: Medical Genetics Knowledge Base. [database online] University of Washington, Seattle. Available at http://www.geneclinics.org

Volpe JJ. Brain injury in the premature infant-neuropathology, clinical aspects, pathogenesis and prevention. Clin Perinatol 1997;24:567–587.

Volpe JJ. Neurology of the Newborn, 4th edn. Philadelphia: WB Saunders, 2001;185–186.

Wyatt JS. Magnetic resonance spectroscopy and near-infrared spectroscopy in the assessment of the asphyxiated term infant. Mental Retard Develop Disabil Res Rev 1997;3:42–48.

3
Hypotonia, Arthrogryposis, and Rigidity

Gerald M. Fenichel

Depressed postural tone is one of the more common neonatal abnormalities requiring neurological consultation. Because normal postural tone requires the integrated functioning of the entire nervous system, depressed postural tone may result from disturbances in either the central or peripheral nervous system (Table 3–1).

Hypotonic newborns look very much the same whether the site of abnormality is in the skeletal muscle or the brain. Chapter 1 includes a description of the characteristic position at rest and the method of testing. Dislocation of the hips is a concomitant feature of antepartum hypotonia. Formation of a normal hip joint requires that the surrounding muscles pull the femoral head into the acetabulum. When muscle tone is depressed, joint cavity formation is retarded and dislocation ensues.

Arthrogryposis, the fixation of joints at birth, is another feature of some newborns with intrauterine hypotonia (Fig. 3–1). Clubfoot is the most frequent deformity, but symmetrical flexion deformities may be present in all limb joints. Contractures in arthrogryposis are probably the nonspecific consequence of intrauterine immobilization. This explanation is not fully satisfactory because, among the several causes of intrauterine immobilization, some disorders regularly produce arthrogryposis and others never do. The differential diagnosis is much the same as for neonatal hypotonia except that extra fetal factors, such as oligohydramnios are also a consideration (Table 3–2). In some newborns with arthrogryposis, no cause can be determined and the contractures resolve spontaneously.

TABLE 3–1   Differential diagnosis of infantile hypotonia

Cerebral hypotonia
1. Benign congenital hypotonia
2. Chronic nonprogressive encephalopathy
   A. Cerebral malformation (see Ch. 8)
   B. Perinatal distress (see Ch. 4)
   C. Postnatal disorders
3. Chromosomal disorders
   A. Autosomal abnormalities
   B. Prader–Willi syndrome
4. Peroxisomal disorders
   A. Cerebrohepatorenal syndrome (Zellweger)
   B. Neonatal adrenoleukodystrophy
5. Other metabolic defects (see Ch. 7)
   A. Acid maltase deficiency
   B. Infantile GM_1 gangliosidosis
6. Other genetic defects
   A. Familial dysautonomia
   B. Oculocerebrorenal syndrome (Lowe)

Neonatal spinal cord injury (see Ch. 5)
1. Breech presentation
2. Cephalic presentation

Motor neuron disorders
1. Spinal muscular atrophies
   A. Acute infantile
   B. Chronic infantile
   C. Infantile neuronal degeneration
   D. Neurogenic arthrogryposis
   E. Incontinentia pigmenti
2. Congenital hypomyelinating neuropathy

Disorders of neuromuscular transmission
1. Infantile botulism
2. Myasthenia gravis
   A. Transitory neonatal myasthenia
   B. Congenital myasthenia
   C. Familial infantile myasthenia

Fiber type disproportion myopathies
1. Congenital fiber type disproportion myopathy
2. Myotubular (centronuclear) myopathy
   A. Acute
   B. Chronic
3. Nemaline (rod) myopathy
4. Central core disease

Muscular dystrophies
1. Congenital muscular dystrophy
   A. Without cerebral involvement
      (i)   Mild
      (ii) Severe
      (iii) Hypotonic-sclerotic

B. With cerebral involvement
    (i)   Fukuyama type
    (ii) With hypomyelination
    (iii) With cerebro-ocular anomalies
C. With autosomal dominant inheritance
2. Myotonic dystrophy

Metabolic myopathies
1. Acid maltase deficiency
2. Cytochrome-*c*-oxidase deficiency
3. Carnitine deficiency
4. Phosphofructokinase deficiency
5. Phosphorylase deficiency

Infantile myositis

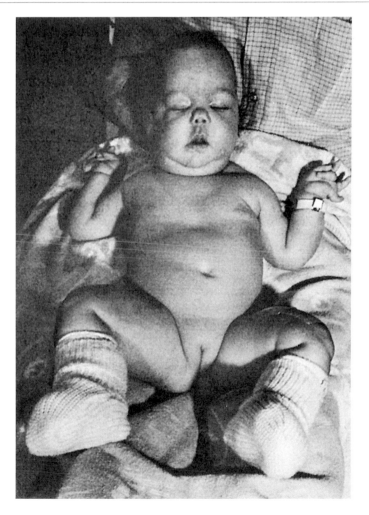

FIGURE 3–1 Arthrogryposis multiplex congenita. Symmetrical flexion deformities are present in all limbs. The mandible is underdeveloped.

TABLE 3–2   Differential diagnosis of arthrogryposis

Non-fetal causes
Fetal, non-nervous system causes
Cerebral malformations
Chromosomal disorders
Cerebrohepatorenal syndrome
Motor unit disorders
   Congenital cervical spinal atrophy
   Congenital fiber type disproportion myopathy
   Congenital muscular dystrophy
   Familial infantile myasthenia
   Infantile neuronal degeneration
   Myotonic dystrophy
   Neurogenic arthrogryposis
   Phosphofructokinase deficiency
   Transitory neonatal myasthenia
X-linked distal arthrogryposis

DIAGNOSTIC APPROACH IN HYPOTONIA

The first step in differential diagnosis is to determine the site of pathology: cerebral, spinal, or motor unit. More than one site may be involved as when muscle weakness impairs respiration and causes postpartum asphyxia, when the underlying disease process affects both the central and peripheral nervous system, and when a difficult delivery has resulted in trauma to the brain, spinal cord, and brachial plexus (Table 3–3). These situations of combined central and peripheral dysfunction often result in delayed diagnosis of one component, despite early diagnosis of the other.

   Cerebral hypotonia is useful as an all-inclusive term for hypotonia due to any encephalopathy. It is the most common cause of hypotonia in the newborn and probably accounts for more than 90% of cases. Most newborns with cerebral hypotonia do not pose a diagnostic dilemma. History and physical examination allow ready identification. Table 3–4 summarizes clues to the diagnosis of cerebral hypotonia. The regular use of computed tomography (CT), magnetic resonance imaging (MRI), and ultrasound (US) in the nursery has significantly improved diagnosis in this group.

TABLE 3–3   Combined cerebral and motor unit hypotonia

Acid maltase deficiency
Familial dysautonomia
Infantile neuronal degeneration
Lipid storage diseases
Mitochondrial disorders
Neonatal myotonic dystrophy
Perinatal asphyxia secondary to motor unit disease

TABLE 3–4   Clues to cerebral hypotonia

Abnormalities of other brain function
Dysmorphic features
Malformations of other organs
Fisting of the hands
Scissoring on vertical suspension
Movement through postural reflexes
Normal or brisk tendon reflexes

Cervical myelopathies are an infrequent cause of hypotonia. The history and examination are the basis for suspecting the diagnosis. MRI often confirms the clinical impression.

A disorder of the motor unit is suggested when the newborn is mentally alert but profoundly weak and areflexic (Table 3–5). Useful studies to refine the diagnosis are the serum creatine kinase (CK) concentration, electromyography (EMG), nerve conduction velocity (NCV) studies, muscle biopsy, and DNA-based testing. Increased serum concentrations of CK are a reflection of skeletal or cardiac muscle necrosis. However, interpreting serum CK requires caution in the newborn, as the concentration is normally high after a vaginal birth and tends to increase during the first 24 hours. Total CK activity and isoenzyme activity increase significantly with acidosis. Levels as high as 1000 IU/L are measured in severely asphyxiated newborns. EMG is useful to select infants for muscle biopsy and has its greatest value in the diagnosis of spinal muscular atrophies and congenital myopathies. Muscle biopsy has its greatest value in the diagnosis of congenital myopathies and dystrophies. DNA-based diagnosis has become the method of choice for the definitive diagnosis of spinal muscular atrophy and some dystrophies.

CEREBRAL HYPOTONIA

Cerebral Hypotonia with Acute Encephalopathy

Hypotonia is a constant feature of acute encephalopathies in all age groups. The differential diagnosis in the newborn is summarized in Table 3–1 and is detailed in other chapters. All acute encephalopathies cause generalized cerebral dysfunction

TABLE 3–5   Clues to motor unit disorders

No abnormalities of other organs
Absent or depressed tendon reflexes
Muscle atrophy
Fasciculations
Failure of movement on postural reflexes

because of edema, inflammation, or hemorrhage. States of decreased consciousness are invariably associated with the hypotonia, and seizures may be present as well. During the acute phase, the tendon reflexes are unobtainable, and the Moro reflex is depressed. As the encephalopathy clears, postural tone remains depressed, but tendon reflexes are obtainable and ankle clonus is common. The Moro reflex is re-established, and jitteriness observed.

The outcome for the child depends directly on the underlying process. In general, muscle tone tends to improve with time. The diagnostic category used to describe infants who were hypotonic at birth and later recovered normal tone is *benign congenital hypotonia*. The term is retrospective and not applicable to the newborn. In many such infants, the cause of the original hypotonia was an acute encephalopathy that later resolved. Despite the recovery of normal muscle tone, an increased incidence of mental retardation, learning disabilities, and other sequelae of cerebral stress are evident later in life. In others, the cause either is a mild myopathy or not established.

Cerebral Hypotonia with Chronic Encephalopathy

Cerebral dysgenesis is the main cause of neonatal hypotonia secondary to chronic encephalopathies. Noxious environmental agents, chromosomal disorders, or genetic defects may cause the dysgenesis (see Table 3–1). All autosomal chromosomal disorders are associated with neonatal hypotonia. Depressed states of consciousness may not be associated unless increased intracranial pressure, inflammation, or seizures are present. The tendon reflexes are brisk at birth, and sustained ankle clonus elicited. Minor stimulation provokes an exaggerated Moro reflex with repeated spreading and clutching movements in the arms. The tonic neck reflex is stereotyped and obligatory, a significant sign of cerebral hemisphere dysfunction. As the head turns from side to side, limbs, that seemed flaccid at rest, develop extension and flexion postures that remain fixed for as long as the head is turned.

Chromosomal Disorders

The number and variety of chromosomal aberrations responsible for human malformation are continually expanding. Despite considerable syndrome diversity in infancy and childhood, the triad of intrauterine growth retardation (IUGR), hypotonia, and anomalies of the face and hands is a reasonably constant feature in the newborn. Hypotonia is present at birth, even when normal tone or spasticity develops later. Arthrogryposis, by itself, is rarely associated with chromosomal aberrations. Even the combination of arthrogryposis and mental retardation carries only a 16% risk of an underlying chromosomal abnormality.

Any hypotonic newborn with 'dysmorphic' features deserves a chromosome study. Even with normal chromosomes, hypotonia in a dysmorphic child is usually due to cerebral dysgenesis. Newborns with hypotonia and dysmorphic features require cranial MRI to determine the extent of cerebral malformation. This information may be useful in therapeutic planning, especially when life-threatening malformations in other organs are present.

Prader–Willi Syndrome Hypotonia, hypogonadism, mental retardation, short stature, and obesity characterize Prader–Willi syndrome. Approximately 70% of children with this syndrome have an interstitial deletion of the paternally contributed proximal long arm of chromosome 15(q11–13) (Cassidy and Schwartz, 2004). The basis for the syndrome in most patients who do not have a deletion is *maternal disomy* (both chromosomes 15 are from the mother). Paternal disomy of chromosome 15 causes *Angelman syndrome.*

- **Clinical features.** Decreased fetal movement occurs in 75% of pregnancies, hip dislocation in 10%, and clubfoot in 6%. Hypotonia is profound at birth and tendon reflexes are absent or greatly depressed. Feeding problems are invariable, and prolonged nasogastric tube feeding is common. Cryptorchidism is present in 84% and hypogenitalism in 100%. However, some newborns lack the associated features and only show hypotonia (Miller et al., 1999).

  Both hypotonia and feeding difficulty persist until 8 to 11 months of age and then replaced by relatively normal muscle tone and insatiable hunger. Delayed developmental milestones and later mental retardation are constant features. Minor abnormalities that become more obvious during infancy include a narrow bifrontal diameter of the skull, strabismus, almond-shaped eyes, enamel hypoplasia, and small hands and feet. Obesity is the rule during childhood. The combination of obesity and minor abnormalities of the face and limbs produces a resemblance among children with this syndrome.

  Major and minor clinical criteria are established (Table 3–6). For children under three years of age, five points are required for diagnosis, four of which must be major criteria. For individuals three years of age and older, eight points are required for diagnosis, at least five of which must be major criteria. Supportive findings only increase or decrease the level of suspicion of the diagnosis.
- **Diagnosis.** DNA-based *methylation* testing detects the absence of the paternally contributed region on *chromosome* 15q11.2–q13 associated with the Prader–Willi syndrome.
- **Management.** Dietary supervision helps control obesity. Specific treatment is not available.

Genetic Disorders

Familial dysautonomia Familial dysautonomia is a genetic disorder transmitted by autosomal recessive inheritance in Ashkenazi Jews. Mutations of an inhibitor of a kinase complex associated protein (IKBKAP) that maps to chromosome 9q31 accounts for almost all cases (Shohat, 2005). Similar clinical syndromes also occur in non-Jewish infants. These are often sporadic and without a known pattern of inheritance. The development and survival of sensory,

TABLE 3–6   Criteria for the clinical diagnosis of Prader–Willi syndrome

Major criteria
Neonatal and infantile central hypotonia with poor suck and improvement with age
Feeding problems and/or failure to thrive in infancy, with need for gavage or other special feeding techniques
Onset of rapid weight gain between 12 months and six years of age, causing central obesity
Hyperphagia
Characteristic facial features: narrow bifrontal diameter, almond-shaped palpebral fissures, down-turned mouth
Hypogonadism:
Genital hypoplasia: small labia minora and clitoris in females; hypoplastic scrotum and cryptorchidism in males
Incomplete and delayed puberty
Infertility
Developmental delay/mild to moderate mental retardation/multiple learning disabilities

Minor criteria
Decreased fetal movement and infantile lethargy, improving with age
Typical behavior problems, including temper tantrums, obsessive-compulsive behavior, stubbornness, rigidity, stealing, and lying
Sleep disturbance/sleep apnea
Short stature for the family by 15 years of age
Hypopigmentation
Small hands and feet for height age
Narrow hands with straight ulnar border
Esotropia, myopia
Thick, viscous saliva
Speech articulation defects
Skin picking

Supportive findings
High pain threshold
Decreased vomiting
Scoliosis and/or kyphosis
Early adrenarche
Osteoporosis
Unusual skill with jigsaw puzzles
Normal neuromuscular studies (e.g. muscle biopsy, EMG, NCV)

From Gunay-Aygun et al. The changing purpose of Prader-Willi syndrome clinical diagnostic criteria and proposed revised criteria. Pediatrics 2001;108:E92.

sympathetic, and parasympathetic neurons are impaired and neuronal degeneration continues throughout childhood.

- **Clinical features.** The important clinical features in affected newborns are meconium aspiration, poor or no sucking reflex, and hypotonia. The causes of hypotonia are disturbances in the brain, the dorsal root ganglia, and the peripheral nerves. Tendon reflexes are hypoactive or absent. The feeding difficulty is unusual and provides a diagnostic clue. Sucking and swallowing are normal separately but cannot be coordinated for effective feeding. Other noticeable clinical features of the newborn or infants are pallor, temperature instability, absent fungiform papillae of the tongue, diarrhea, and abdominal distention. Poor weight gain and lethargy, episodic irritability, absent corneal reflexes, labile blood pressure, and failure to produce overflow tears completes the clinical picture.

- **Diagnosis.** Ophthalmological examination is useful to detect the signs of postganglionic parasympathetic denervation: supersensitivity of the pupil, shown by a positive miotic response to 0.1% pilocarpine or 2.5% methacholine, corneal insensitivity, and absence of tears. Targeted mutation analysis to establish the diagnosis is commercially available.
- **Management.** Improved supportive treatment has extended survival and 60% of affected children reaching 20 years of age (Axelrod et al., 2002). Pulmonary disease and sepsis are significant causes of death. Management of feeding problems in the newborn includes adequate nutrition with avoidance of aspiration, prevention of aspiration, and daily chest physiotherapy. Management of orthostatic hypotension includes hydration and fludrocortisone. Decreased corneal sensation and absence of tearing requires the use of artificial tear solutions.

Oculocerebrorenal Syndrome (Lowe syndrome)   Reduced activity of the enzyme inositol polyphosphate 5-phosphatase (OCRL-1) is the cause of the syndrome. The responsible gene locus is at Xq26.1. Inheritance is X-linked recessive (Wappner, 2003).

- **Clinical features.** The important features in affected male newborns are hypotonia and hyporeflexia, sometimes associated with congenital cataracts and glaucoma. Features that appear later in infancy are mental retardation and a progressive disorder of the renal tubules resulting in metabolic acidosis, proteinuria, aminoaciduria, and defective acidification of the urine. Many infants die after failing to thrive. Others have mild symptoms, including growth retardation, borderline intellectual function, mild renal disturbances, and late-onset cataract formation. Life expectancy is normal in the milder cases.
    Carrier females are normal at birth but may develop cataracts in adolescence.
- **Diagnosis.** Diagnosis depends on recognition of the clinical constellation. MRI shows diffuse and irregular foci of increased signal consistent with demyelination. OCRL-1 activity is measurable in cultured fibroblasts. Molecular genetic testing is available for carrier detection.
- **Management.** Most patients require alkalization therapy, and many benefit from supplements of potassium, phosphate, calcium, and carnitine.

Peroxisomal Disorders   Peroxisomes are subcellular organelles that participate in the biosynthesis of ether phospholipids and bile acids; the oxidation of very-long-chain fatty acids (VLCFA), prostaglandins, and unsaturated long-chain fatty acids; and the catabolism of phytanate, pipecolate, and glycolate. Hydrogen peroxide is a product of several oxidation reactions, and catabolized by the enzyme catalase. Mutations in eleven different PEX genes cause this spectrum of disorders. PEX genes encode the proteins required for peroxisomal assembly.

The infantile syndromes of peroxisomal dysfunction are all disorders of peroxisomal biogenesis; the intrinsic protein membrane is identifiable, but all matrix enzymes are missing. The prototype, cerebrohepatorenal (Zellweger) syndrome (ZS), is a continuum of phenotypes that include neonatal adrenoleukodystrophy and infantile Refsum disease (see Ch. 16). The latter are milder variants. Infantile hypotonia is a prominent feature of peroxisomal biogenesis disorders (Steinberg et al., 2003).

MOTOR NEURON DISEASES

Motor neuron diseases are a heterogeneous group of disorders, usually genetic in origin, characterized by the degeneration of anterior horn cells in the spinal cord and of motor nuclei in the brainstem. Some of these disorders have a localized distribution (Moebius syndrome and congenital cervical spinal atrophy) while others are generalized. The most prominent member of this group in newborns is infantile spinal muscular atrophy (SMA).

Spinal Muscular Atrophy

The severe type (SMA I) always begins before six months. The SMN1 (survival motor neuron) gene on chromosome 5q12.2–q13.3 is the primary SMA disease-causing gene (Prior and Russman, 2003). Normal individuals have both the SMN1 gene and the SMN2 gene, an almost identical copy of the SMN1 gene, on the same chromosome.

- **Clinical features.** The age at onset is birth to 6 months. Reduced fetal movement may occur when neuronal degeneration begins in utero. Affected newborns have generalized weakness involving proximal more than distal muscles, hypotonia, and areflexia. Newborns that are hypotonic in utero and weak at birth may have difficulty adapting to extrauterine life and experience postnatal asphyxia and encephalopathy. Most breathe adequately at first and appear alert despite the generalized weakness because facial expression is relatively well preserved and extraocular movement is normal. Some newborns have paradoxical respiration because intercostal paralysis and thoracic collapse occur before diaphragmatic movement is impaired, while others have diaphragmatic paralysis as an initial feature. Despite intrauterine hypotonia, arthrogryposis is not present. Neurogenic arthrogryposis may be a distinct entity and described separately in this chapter.
- **Diagnosis.** Molecular genetic testing of the SMN1 gene is available. About 95% of individuals with SMA are homozygous for the absence of exon 7 and 8 of SMN1 and about 5% are compound heterozygotes for absence of exons 7 and 8 of SMN1 and a point mutation in SMN1. The serum concentration of CK is usually normal but may be mildly elevated in infants with rapidly progressive weakness. EMG studies show fibrillations and

fasciculations at rest, and the mean amplitude of motor unit potentials is increased. Motor nerve conduction velocities are usually normal.

Muscle biopsy is often unnecessary because of the commercial availability of DNA-based testing. The pathological findings in skeletal muscle are characteristic. Routine histological stains show groups of small fibers adjacent to groups of normal-sized or hypertrophied fibers. When the myosin ATPase reaction is applied, all hypertrophied fibers are type I, whereas medium-sized and small fibers are a mixture of types I and II (Fig. 3–2). Type grouping, a sign of reinnervation in which large numbers of fibers of the same type are contiguous, replaces the normal random arrangement of fiber types. Some biopsy specimens show uniform small fibers of both types.

- **Management.** Treatment is supportive. DNA analysis of chorion villus biopsies provides prenatal diagnosis.

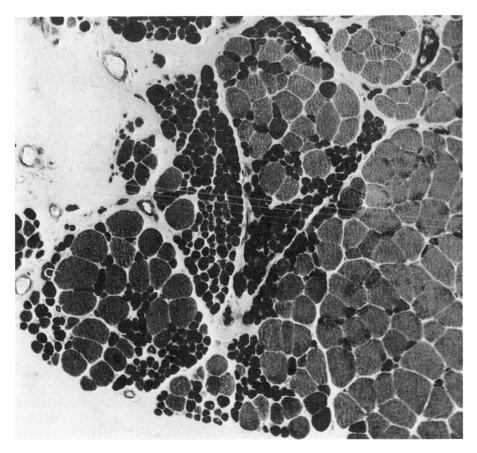

FIGURE 3–2 Infantile spinal muscular atrophy (ATPase). The normal checkerboard pattern is lost. Groups of large type I fibers are adjacent to groups of small type II fibers.

Infantile Spinal Muscular Atrophy with Respiratory Distress Type 1 (SMARD1)

Originally classified as a variant of SMA1, SMARD1 is a distinct genetic disorder resulting from mutations in the gene encoding the immunoglobulin μ-binding protein 2 (IGHMBP2) on chromosome 11q13 (Grohmann et al., 2003).

- **Clinical features.** Intrauterine growth retardation, weak cry, and foot deformities are the initial features. Most infants come to attention between 1 and 6 months because of respiratory distress secondary to diaphragmatic weakness, weak cry, and progressive distal weakness of the legs. Sensory and autonomic nerve dysfunction accompanies the motor weakness. Sudden infant death occurs without respiratory support.
- **Diagnosis.** Consider the diagnosis in infants with a SMA-1 phenotype lacking the 5q gene abnormality, and those with distal weakness and respiratory failure.
- **Management.** Treatment is supportive.

Neurogenic Arthrogryposis

The original use of the term neurogenic arthrogryposis was to denote the association of arthrogryposis with infantile spinal muscular atrophy. Transmission occurs by autosomal recessive inheritance in some families and by X-linked inheritance in others. Some individuals with autosomal recessive inheritance have deletions in the SMN gene. I am aware of two sets of identical twins in which one twin was born with neurogenic arthrogryposis and the other remained normal. This suggests that some cases may have nongenetic causes.

Families with X-linked neurogenic arthrogryposis tend to have clinical or pathological features that distinguish them from others. Arthrogryposis may not occur in every affected family member, weakness or joint deformity may be limited to the legs or arms, and progression is minimal.

- **Clinical features.** In neurogenic arthrogryposis, the most active phase of disease occurs in utero. Severely affected newborns have respiratory and feeding difficulties, and some die of aspiration. The less severely affected ones survive and have little or no progression of their weakness. Indeed, the respiratory and feeding difficulties lessen with time. Contractures are present in both proximal and distal joints. Micrognathia and a high-arched palate may be associated features, and a pattern of facial anomalies suggesting trisomy 18 is present in some newborns. Newborns with respiratory distress at birth may not have a fatal course. Limb weakness may be minimal, and long intervals of stability occur.
- **Diagnosis.** Suspect the diagnosis in newborns with arthrogryphosis, normal serum concentrations of CK, and EMG findings compatible with a neuropathic process. Muscle histological examination reveals the typical pattern of denervation and reinnervation. Cranial MRI investigates cerebral malformations in children with microcephaly.

- **Management.** Initiate an intensive program of rehabilitation immediately after birth. Surgical release of contractures is often required.

Moebius Syndrome

A typical Moebius syndrome is congenital palsy of lateral gaze and facial expression secondary to agenesis of cranial nerves VI and VII. Generalized hypotonia may be present as well. The syndrome appears to be a restricted form of motor neuron disease with primary involvement of cranial nerve nuclei. The lack of progressive weakness suggests that the basic pathology is an agenesis of neurons rather than an intrauterine atrophy.

- **Clinical features.** The Moebius syndrome is the best-known congenital aplasia of facial nerve nuclei and facial muscles. The site of pathology is usually the facial nerve nuclei and their internuclear connections. Facial diplegia may occur alone, with bilateral abducens palsies, or with involvement of several cranial nerves (Harriette et al., 2003). Congenital malformations elsewhere in the body—dextrocardia, talipes equinovarus, absent pectoral muscle, and limb deformities—are sometimes associated features. Most cases are sporadic, but familial recurrence occurs. Autosomal dominant, autosomal recessive and X-linked recessive modes of inheritance are proposed. Identified loci are on chromosome 13, 3, and 10.
- **Diagnosis.** The clinical features establish the diagnosis.
- **Management.** Treatment is supportive.

CERVICAL MYELOPATHIES

Transection of the cervical cord is a rare consideration in the differential diagnosis of neonatal hypotonia because the clinical features are not sufficiently specific to divert attention from other pathological entities that occur with greater frequency. It is only by vigilance to the possibility of cervical myelopathy that one minimizes time and expense in the diagnostic evaluation. The discussion of physical injury, the most common cause of cervical myelopathy, is in Chapter 5. Cervical myelomeningocele is exceptionally uncommon and is not ordinarily part of the differential diagnosis of neonatal hypotonia because of the obvious dorsal defect. Chapter 8 considers dysraphic states.

Congenital Atlantoaxial Dislocation

The odontoid process, in position between the anterior ring of the atlas ventrally and the transverse ligament dorsally, is the main structure preventing dislocation of C1 on C2. Maldevelopment of the odontoid process or the transverse ligament results in congenital atlantoaxial dislocation and cervical myelopathy. Aplasia of the odontoid process can occur alone or as part of Morquio syndrome, other mucopolysaccharidoses, Klippel–Feil syndrome, several types of genetic chondrodysplasia, and some chromosomal abnormalities.

- **Clinical features.** The primary feature of the myelopathy resulting from atlantoaxial dislocation is an acute or slowly progressive quadriplegia, which usually begins during childhood or young adult life. When the onset is in the newborn, the clinical picture resembles SMA-I. Hypotonia, while generalized, spares facial expression and extraocular movement. Tendon reflexes are at first absent but later become hyperactive. Sustained ankle clonus is present.
- **Diagnosis.** The first clue to the diagnosis of congenital atlantoaxial dislocation is the recording of a normal EMG in a newborn who appears to have SMA-I. Lateral radiographs of the cervical portion of the spine in extension and flexion may show atlantoaxial instability, but CT of the cervical vertebrae provides better documentation of the instability and of the spinal cord compression. When suspecting Morquio syndrome, check the urine for keratan sulfate.
- **Management.** The goal of treatment is reduction of the dislocation and fixation of the vertebrae. Subsequent recovery of function is variable and depends upon the degree of pre-existing spinal cord damage.

POLYNEUROPATHY

Symptomatic polyneuropathies are exceptionally rare in the newborn period. In some leukodystrophies (metachromatic and globoid), electrophysiological, but not clinical, evidence of neuropathy is present early in infancy. Among the many disorders that cause polyneuropathy in infancy and childhood, only congenital hypomyelinating neuropathy has a neonatal onset.

Congenital Hypomyelinating Neuropathy

- **Clinical features.** The symptoms and signs in the newborn are indistinguishable from acute infantile spinal muscular atrophy. Hypotonia is present at birth accompanied by arthrogryposis of one or more limbs. Respiratory failure may require ventilatory support. Other features may include facial diplegia and arthrogryposis.

    Progressive flaccid weakness, skeletal muscle atrophy, and bulbar weakness sparing extraocular motility follows. Respiratory insufficiency causes death during infancy. Peripheral nerves enlarge and may become palpable when survival is prolonged (Szigeti et al., 2003).
- **Diagnosis.** Motor nerve conduction velocity slows and sural nerve biopsy shows little or no compact myelin and few onion bulbs. Genetic analysis detects mutations in the myelin protein zero gene.
- **Management.** Treatment is supportive.

DISORDERS OF NEUROMUSCULAR TRANSMISSION

Botulism

Human botulism ordinarily results from eating food contaminated by preformed exotoxin of the organism *Clostridium botulinum*. The exotoxin prevents the release of acetylcholine, causing a cholinergic blockade of skeletal muscle and end organs innervated by autonomic nerves. Infantile botulism is an age-limited disorder in which ingested *C. botulinum* colonizes the intestinal tract, and produces toxin in situ. This can only occur in newborns and young infants because competing organisms have not yet colonized the intestinal tract. Dietary contamination with honey or corn syrup accounts for almost 20% of cases, but in most the source is not defined (Cherington, 1998). Few cases have occurred during the newborn period and always after discharge from the nursery to home.

- **Clinical features.** The clinical spectrum of infantile botulism includes (1) asymptomatic carriers of organisms; (2) mild hypotonia and failure to thrive; (3) severe, progressive, life-threatening paralysis; (4) and sudden infant death. A distinct seasonal incidence occurs between March and October. In severe cases, constipation and poor feeding occur first and are followed within 4 to 5 days by a progressive bulbar and skeletal muscle weakness and loss of tendon reflexes that suggests the Guillain–Barré syndrome or SMA-I. Botulism differentiates clinically from SMA by the early appearance of facial and pharyngeal weakness; the presence of ptosis and dilated pupils that respond sluggishly or not at all to light; and the occurrence of severe constipation or diarrhea.
- **Diagnosis.** EMG readily distinguishes botulism from SMA and the Guillain–Barré syndrome. Repetitive stimulation between 20 and 50 stimuli per second reverses the presynaptic block and produces an incremental increase in the size of the motor unit potentials in 90% of cases. The EMG shows short-duration, low-amplitude motor unit potentials. Isolation of toxin and/or organism from the stool confirms the diagnosis.
- **Management.** Infantile botulism is a self-limited disease generally lasting 2 to 6 weeks. The use of antitoxin and antibiotics does not influence its course. Indeed, gentamicin, an agent that produces presynaptic neuromuscular blockade, may worsen the condition. Intensive care is required throughout the period of profound hypotonia, and many infants require respiratory support. Sudden apnea and death are a constant danger.

Transitory Neonatal Myasthenia

Ten to twenty percent of children born to myasthenic mothers develop a transitory myasthenic syndrome (Hoff et al., 2003). The syndrome is probably secondary to the passive transfer of antibody directed against fetal AChR from the myasthenic mother to her normal fetus. Fetal AChR is structurally different from adult AChR. The severity of symptoms in the newborn correlates with the ratio of fetal to adult AChR antibodies in the mother but does not correlate with the severity or duration of weakness in the mother.

- **Clinical features.** Woman with myasthenia have a higher rate of complications of delivery (Hoff et al., 2003). Difficulty feeding and generalized hypotonia are the major clinical features in the infant. Affected children are eager to feed, but the ability to suck fatigues quickly and nutrition is inadequate. Symptoms usually arise within hours of birth but delay until the third day occurs. Some newborns were hypotonic in utero and born with arthrogryposis. Weakness of cry and lack of facial expression is present in 50%, but only 15% have limitation of extraocular movement and ptosis. Respiratory insufficiency is uncommon. Weakness becomes progressively worse in the first few days and then improves. The mean duration of symptoms is 18 days, with a range of 5 days to 2 months. Recovery is complete, and transitory neonatal myasthenia does not develop into myasthenia gravis later in life.
- **Diagnosis.** The diagnosis of transitory neonatal myasthenia requires temporary reversal of weakness following subcutaneous or intravenous injection of edrophonium chloride, 0.15 mg/kg.
- **Management.** Plasma exchange treats newborns with severe generalized weakness and respiratory distress. For those who are less impaired, an intramuscular injection of 0.1% neostigmine methylsulfate before feeding sufficiently improves sucking and swallowing to allow adequate nutrition. Progressively reduce the dose as symptoms remit. Nasogastric tube administration of neostigmine requires a dose 10 times the parenteral level.

Genetic Myasthenias

Several genetic defects causing myasthenic syndromes have been identified (Table 3–7). All are autosomal recessive traits except for the slow channel syndrome, which is an autosomal dominant trait (see Ch. 7). Among the autosomal recessive forms, the causative mutation in one is in the choline acetyltransferase gene on chromosome 10q and another that maps to chromosome 17. All genetic myasthenic syndromes are seronegative for antibodies that bind the acetylcholine

TABLE 3–7   Genetic forms of myasthenia gravis

Presynaptic defects
1. Abnormal ACh resynthesis or mobilization
2. Paucity of synaptic vesicles and reduced quantal release. Abnormal ACh release

Postsynaptic defects
1. Endplate AChE deficiency
2. Kinetic abnormalities of the receptor without primary AChR deficiency
3. Abnormal interaction of acetylcholine and receptor
4. High conductance and fast closure of the acetylcholine receptor channel

Slow channel syndrome

receptor (AChR). Both the genetic and clinical features are the basis for classifying congenital myasthenic syndromes.

Few laboratories are able to determine the site of abnormality or the responsible gene. Therefore, clinicians recognize two clinical syndromes: familial infantile myasthenia with prominent respiratory and feeding difficulty at birth, and congenital myasthenia with predominantly ocular findings (see Ch. 15). The causes of familial infantile myasthenia include a presynaptic defect in acetylcholine resynthesis and packaging and several postsynaptic defects involving the kinetics of the AChR or congenital endplate acetylcholinesterase deficiency.

- **Clinical features.** Respiratory insufficiency and feeding difficulty may be present at birth. Many affected newborns require mechanical ventilation. Ptosis and generalized weakness either are present at birth or develop during infancy (Mullaney et al., 2000). Arthrogryposis may also be present. Although facial and skeletal muscles are weak, extraocular motility is usually normal. Within weeks, the infants become stronger and no longer need mechanical ventilation. However, episodes of weakness and life-threatening apnea occur repeatedly throughout infancy and childhood, sometimes even into adult life.
- **Diagnosis.** The intravenous or subcutaneous injection of edrophonium chloride, 0.15 mg/kg establishes the diagnosis. The weakness and the respiratory distress reverse almost immediately after intravenous injection and within 10 minutes of subcutaneous injection. A decrement in the amplitude of successive motor unit potentials with low frequency repetitive nerve stimulation confirms the diagnosis. Identification of the precise defect requires special laboratory techniques.
- **Management.** Long-term treatment with neostigmine or pyridostigmine prevents sudden episodes of apnea at the time of intercurrent illness. The weakness in some children responds to a combination of pyridostigmine and diaminopyridine (DAP). DAP is not commercially available in the United States but can be obtained on a compassionate use basis from Jacobus Pharmaceutical Company, Inc., Princeton, NJ, fax no. 609–799–1176. Thymectomy and immunosuppressive therapy are not beneficial.

CONGENITAL MYOPATHIES

Several 'congenital myopathies' present as neonatal hypotonia and are difficult to distinguish from each other on clinical grounds alone. Cerebral function and sensation are intact unless there is some element of asphyxia, tendon reflexes may be present or absent, and the serum concentration of CK is usually normal. EMG is usually abnormal but not diagnostic. Diagnosis depends entirely upon muscle biopsy. A common finding, when histochemical reactions are applied, is that type I muscle fibers are greater in number (fiber type predominance) but smaller in size than type II muscle fibers (Fig. 3–3). This *fiber type disproportion* is the only histological abnormality in some patients, while in others a unique histological feature is present which identifies the condition. The discussions of

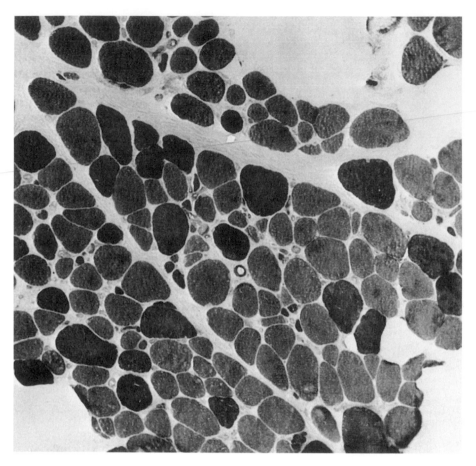

FIGURE 3–3   Fiber type disproportion myopathy (ATPase). Type I fibers are more numerous than type II fibers. The type II fibers are generally larger in diameter than the type I fibers.

myotubular myopathy, nemaline myopathy, and central core disease are in this section. Other 'unique histological features' occur with lesser frequency and are not discussed here.

Congenital Fiber-Type Disproportion Myopathy

The congenital fiber-type disproportion (CFTD) myopathies are a heterogeneous group of diseases that have a similar pattern of muscle histology. The initial feature of all these diseases is infantile hypotonia. Both sexes are involved equally. Most cases are sporadic; some are clearly autosomal dominant traits and others are autosomal recessive. Despite the label 'congenital,' an identical pattern of fiber-type disproportion may be present in patients who are asymptomatic at birth and first have weakness during childhood.

- **Clinical features.** The severity of weakness in the newborn varies from mild hypotonia to respiratory insufficiency. Many had intrauterine hypotonia and show congenital hip dislocation, dysmorphic features, and joint contractures. Proximal muscles are weaker than distal muscles. Facial weakness, high arched palate, ptosis, and disturbances of ocular motility may be present. When axial weakness is present in infancy, kyphoscoliosis often develops during childhood. Tendon reflexes are depressed or absent. Intellectual function is normal. Weakness is most severe during the first 2 years and then becomes relatively stable or progresses slowly.
- **Diagnosis.** The essential feature seen in muscle specimens is type I fiber predominance and hypotrophy. Type I fibers are 15% smaller than type II fibers. Other laboratory studies are not helpful. The serum concentration of CK may be slightly elevated or normal, and the EMG may be consistent with a neuropathic process, a myopathic process, or both. Nerve conduction velocities are normal.
- **Management.** Physical therapy should be initiated immediately, not only to relieve existing contractures but also to prevent new contractures from developing.

Central Core Disease

Central core disease is a rare but distinct genetic entity transmitted by autosomal dominant inheritance. Mutations in the ryanodine receptor-1 gene (RYR1) on chromosome 19q13 are responsible for central core disease and malignant hyperthermia (Monnier et al., 2000).

- **Clinical features.** Mild hypotonia is present immediately after birth or during infancy. Congenital dislocation of the hips is relatively common. Slowly progressive weakness begins after the age of 5 years. Weakness is greater in proximal than in distal limb muscles and is greater in the arms than in the legs. Tendon reflexes of weak muscles are depressed or absent. Extraocular motility, facial expression, and swallowing are normal. Some children become progressively weaker, have motor impairment, and develop kyphoscoliosis. In others, weakness remains mild and never causes disability.

    Most children with central core disease are at risk of malignant hyperthermia and should not be administered anesthetics without appropriate caution (see Ch. 8).
- **Diagnosis.** The serum concentration of CK is normal, and the EMG findings may be normal as well. More frequently, the EMG suggests a myopathic process. Diagnosis depends on muscle biopsy. Sharply demarcated cores of closely packed myofibrils undergoing varying degrees of degeneration are present in the center of all type I fibers (Fig. 3–4). Because of the tight packing of myofibrils, the cores are deficient in sarcoplasmic reticulum, glycogen, and mitochondria.
- **Management.** Treatment is supportive.

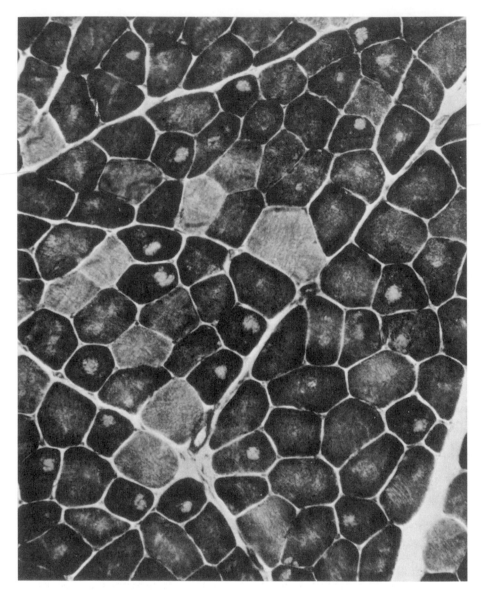

FIGURE 3–4   Myotubular (centronuclear) myopathy (trichrome). A spectrum of muscle fiber sizes is observed. Most fibers have a central nucleus. The small fibers are all type I.

Myotubular (Centronuclear) Myopathy

Several clinical syndromes are included in the category of myotubular (centronuclear) myopathy. Transmission of some is by X-linked inheritance, others by autosomal dominant inheritance, and still others by autosomal recessive inheritance. The autosomal dominant form has a later onset and a milder course. The common histological feature on muscle biopsy is an apparent arrest in the morphogenesis of the muscle fiber at the myotube stage.

Acute Myotubular Myopathy

The abnormal gene that causes acute myotubular myopathy (MTM) maps to the long arm of the X chromosome (Xq28) and is designated MTM1. *Myotubularin* is the protein encoded by the MTM1 gene (Das and Herman, 2004).

- **Clinical features.** Newborns with severe MTM1 are hypotonic and require respiratory assistance. The face is myopathic, motor milestones delayed, and most fail to walk. Death in infancy is common. Those with forms that are more moderate achieve motor milestones more quickly and about 40% require no ventilator support. In the mildest forms, ventilatory support is only required in the newborn period; delay of motor milestones is mild, walking is achieved, and facial strength is normal. Weakness is not progressive and may improve slowly over time. Female *carriers* are generally asymptomatic.
- **Diagnosis.** The serum concentration of CK is normal. The EMG may suggest a neuropathic process, a myopathic process, or both. Muscle biopsy shows type I fiber predominance and hypotrophy, the presence of many internal nuclei, and a central area of increased oxidative enzyme and decreased myosin ATPase activity (Fig. 3.5). Molecular genetic testing is available.
- **Management.** Treatment is supportive.

Chronic Myotubular Myopathy

Inheritance of chronic myotubular myopathy may be either autosomal dominant or recessive inheritance. Some forms are associated with mutations in the myogenic factor-6 gene (12q21).

- **Clinical features.** In general, age at onset of the recessive form is during infancy and ophthalmoplegia is often associated. Mutations in chromosome 12q21 cause the dominant form. Some affected children have hypotonia at birth, but onset in most is during infancy. They come to attention because of delayed motor development. The pattern of limb weakness may be proximal or distal. The axial and neck flexor muscles are weak as well. The course is usually slowly progressive. Possible features include ophthalmoplegia, loss of facial expression, and continuing weakness of limb muscles. Some have seizures and mental deficiency.
- **Diagnosis.** The serum concentration of CK is normal, and EMG findings are abnormal but do not establish the diagnosis. Muscle biopsy is essential for diagnosis, and the histological features are identical to those of the acute form.
- **Management.** Treatment is supportive.

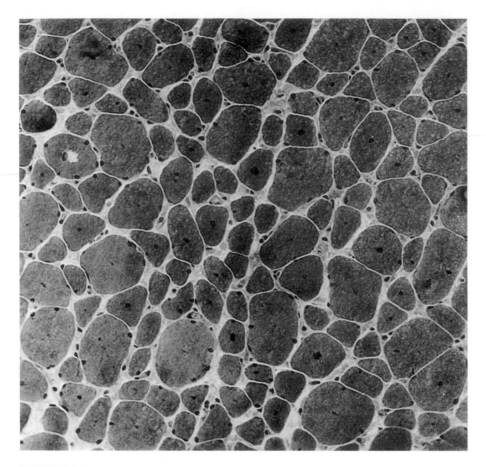

FIGURE 3–5   Nemaline (rod) myopathy (trichrome). A spectrum of fiber sizes is present. The small fibers are all type I and contain rod-like bodies in a subsarcolemmal position.

Nemaline (Rod) Myopathy

Transmission of nemaline myopathy is either as an autosomal dominant or recessive trait. Approximately 20% of cases are recessive, 30% dominant, and 50% sporadic (North, 2002). Several different genetic abnormalities cause the same histological features that define the disorder.

- **Clinical features.** Nemaline myopathy (NM) is characterized by weakness and hypotonia with depressed or absent deep tendon reflexes. Muscle weakness is usually most severe in the face, the neck flexors, and the proximal limb muscles. Significant differences exist in survival between patients classified as having severe, intermediate, and typical *congenital* NM. The severity of neonatal respiratory disease and the presence of arthrogryposis multiplex congenita are associated with death in the first year of life. Independent ambulation before 18 months of age is predictive of survival. Most children with typical congenital NM are eventually able to walk.

At least three different phenotypes occur in children. Transmission of two congenital types is by autosomal recessive inheritance: (1) a severe neonatal form that causes immediate respiratory insufficiency and neonatal death and (2) a milder form in which affected newborns often appear normal or are mildly hypotonic and not brought to medical attention until motor milestones are delayed. This form tends to be slowly progressive, with greater weakness in proximal than distal muscles. Weakness of facial muscles causes a dysmorphic appearance in which the face appears long and narrow and the palate is high and arched. Axial weakness leads to scoliosis.

Transmission of the childhood-onset form is by autosomal dominant inheritance. Onset of ankle weakness occurs late in the first or early in the second decade. The weakness is slowly progressive, and affected individuals may be wheelchair confined as adults.

- **Diagnosis.** The serum concentration of CK is either normal or only mildly elevated. EMG findings may be normal, and when abnormal they are not the basis for diagnosis. Muscle biopsy is essential for diagnosis. Within most fibers are multiple small rod-like particles, thought derived from lateral expansion of the Z disk. The greatest concentration of particles is under the sarcolemma (Fig. 3–6). Type I fiber predominance is a prominent feature. Molecular diagnosis is available for the *alpha actin gene* (ACT1) responsible for both congenital and childhood forms.
- **Management.** Treatment is supportive. Parents who have the abnormal gene but are not weak may have rod bodies and fiber-type predominance in their muscles.

CONGENITAL DYSTROPHINOPATHY

Dystrophinopathies usually have their onset in childhood as Duchenne or Becker muscular dystrophy. Sometimes they cause weakness at birth or enlarged, indurated limb muscles secondary to rhabdomyolysis. In cases with neonatal onset, dystrophin is completely absent. The serum CK concentration is markedly elevated. Immunofluorescence reactions for all three domains of dystrophin show no reactivity.

CONGENITAL MUSCULAR DYSTROPHY

The congenital muscular dystrophies (CMD) are a group of myopathies characterized by hypotonia at birth or shortly thereafter, the early formation of multiple joint contractures, and diffuse muscle weakness and atrophy (Gordon et al., 2005).

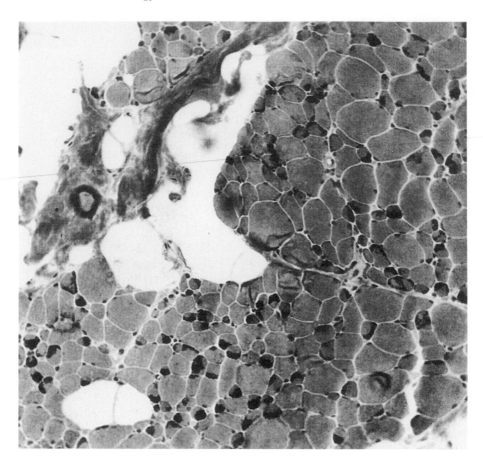

FIGURE 3–6 Central core disease (DPNH). A central area devoid of mitochondrial enzyme activity is observed in most type I fibers. (Courtesy of Dr Michael Brooke.)

Inheritance of all CMD is autosomal recessive. CMD are divisible into syndromic and nonsyndromic forms. In syndromic CMD, both muscle and brain are abnormal. In nonsyndromic forms, muscular disease occurs without cerebral involvement.

An alternative classification of CMD is by the absence or presence of *merosin* (laminin a$_2$) in muscle. Merosin, located in the extracellular matrix, is the linking protein for the dystroglycan complex. Merosin-deficiency may be primary or secondary. Primary merosin deficiency only affects muscle while secondary merosin deficiencies occur in the syndromic CMD.

The congenital muscular dystrophies are genetic disturbances of structural proteins. As a group, they have a more devastating course than the congenital myopathies.

Nonsyndromic Congenital Muscular Dystrophy

Merosin-Positive Nonsyndromic CMD

The phenotype associated with merosin-positive CMD is not homogeneous. Transmission is by autosomal recessive inheritance with considerable genetic heterogeneity. One form, mapped to chromosome 1p36–p35, consistently shows early rigidity of the spine, scoliosis, and reduced vital capacity, as are found in the *rigid spine syndrome* (Flanigan et al., 2000). *Ullrich disease*, caused by mutations in the collagen VI gene, is a form of CMD in which muscle fibers necrosis is secondary to loss of collagen links (Ishikawa et al., 2002).

- **Clinical features.** Approximately half of affected individuals are abnormal at birth because of some combination of hypotonia, poor ability to suck, and respiratory distress. Delayed achievement of motor milestones is usual. Limb-girdle weakness is the rule, generalized weakness may be present, and about half of the individuals have facial weakness. Joint deformities may be present at birth or develop during infancy.
- **Diagnosis.** The serum concentration of CK is mildly elevated, and muscle biopsy shows fiber necrosis and regeneration. Brain MRI is normal.
- **Management.** Physical therapy is important to prevent and reduce contractures.

Merosin-Deficient Nonsyndromic CMD

The abnormal gene site for primary merosin-deficient CMD is chromosome 6q22–23. The abnormal protein is laminin. The phenotypes associated with merosin deficiency are generally more severe than the phenotypes with merosin present. Merosin deficiency is also associated with later onset muscular dystrophies (Jones et al., 2001).

- **Clinical features.** Hypotonia, arthrogryposis, and respiratory insufficiency are severe at birth. The infant has generalized limb weakness, with proximal muscles affected earlier and more severely than distal muscles. Facial and neck weakness is common, but extraocular motility is normal. Tendon reflexes may be present or absent and are often difficult to test because of joint contractures. Contractures at birth may involve any joint, but torticollis and clubfoot are particularly common, and congenital dislocation of the hips is often an associated feature.

  Muscle hypertrophy is not present. Weakness and contractures delay motor development. The best motor achievement is the ability to sit unsupported. Intelligence is either normal or borderline subnormal. Chronic hypoventilation leading to respiratory failure is the usual cause of death.
- **Diagnosis.** The serum concentration of CK is high in the newborn and tends to decline with age. Asymptomatic siblings and parents may have elevated serum concentrations of CK. EMG findings are consistent with a myopathic process. The muscle histological appearance is characteristic. Features include a variation in fiber size with occasional central nucleation,

extensive fibrosis, and proliferation of adipose tissue, fibers undergoing regeneration and degeneration, and thickening of the muscle spindle capsule. A mononuclear infiltrate surrounding muscle fibers is often present early in the course. Cases of 'neonatal polymyositis' are actually merosin-deficient CMD. Molecular genetic diagnosis is available.

Infants who are merosin deficient have an abnormal T_2 MRI signal in the cerebral white matter indicating hypomyelination mainly in the occipital horns. Structural disturbances of the occipital cortex may be associated (Philpot et al., 1999).

- **Management.** Physical therapy is important to prevent further contractures.

Syndromic Congenital Muscular Dystrophy

In at least four disorders, congenital muscular dystrophy coexists with involvement of the central nervous system. These are *Fukuyama CMD* (FCMD), *muscle–eye–brain disease* (MEBD), the *Walker–Warburg syndrome* (WWS) and *congenital muscular dystrophy type 1D* (MDCID). FCMD occurs almost exclusively in Japan, MEBD occurs mainly in Finland, and WWS has wide geographical distribution. Each has a different gene abnormality. A single case report of MDC1D exists (Longman et al., 2003). The gene has a role in the glycosylation of alpha dystroglycan.

The major feature of the first three is a disturbance of cellular migration to the cortex between the fourth and fifth gestational months, resulting in polymicrogyria, lissencephaly, and heterotopia. Other abnormalities may include fusion of the frontal lobes, hydrocephalus, periventricular cysts, optic nerve atrophy, hypoplasia of the pyramidal tracts, reduction in the number of anterior horn cells, and inflammation of the leptomeninges.

WWS and FCMD show reduced but not absent merosin expression. MEBD has normal merosin expression. An abnormal MRI T_2 signal in the centrum semiovale that resembles hypomyelination is a marker of abnormal merosin expression.

- **Clinical features.** FCMD is the most common form of muscular dystrophy in Japan. One quarter of mothers with an affected child, have a history of spontaneous abortion. Affected newborns are normal at birth but soon develop hypotonia, an expressionless face, a weak cry, and an ineffective suck. Weakness affects proximal more than distal limb muscles. Mild contractures of the elbow and knee joints may be present at birth or develop later. Tendon reflexes are usually absent. Pseudohypertrophy of the calves develops in half of cases. Affected children may achieve sitting balance, but never stand.

  Symptoms of cerebral involvement are present early in infancy. Febrile or nonfebrile generalized seizures are usually the first manifestation. Delayed development is always global and microcephaly is the rule. Mental retardation is severe. Weakness and atrophy are progressive and result in severe disability, cachexia, and death before 10 years of age.

Neonatal hypotonia, developmental delay, and ocular abnormalities characterize MEBD. Most affected children walk by age 4 years and then decline in all psychomotor skills. Specific eye abnormalities include glaucoma, progressive myopia, progressive retinal atrophy, and juvenile cataracts. The cerebral and muscle abnormalities of WWS are similar to those in MEBD. Ocular abnormalities include corneal clouding, cataracts, retinal dysplasia or detachment, and optic nerve hypoplasia.

Characteristics of MDCID is global developmental delay, moderate muscle hypertrophy, mild facial weakness, proximal greater than distal limb weakness, and extensive white matter changes on MRI.

- **Diagnosis.** Molecular genetic testing is available for all syndromes. The serum concentration of CK is generally elevated, and the EMG indicates a myopathy. Muscle biopsy specimens show excessive proliferation of adipose tissue and collagen out of proportion to the degree of fiber degeneration. Typical MRI abnormalities are dilatation of the cerebral ventricles and subarachnoid space and lucency of cortical white matter.
- **Management.** Treatment is supportive.

Congenital Myotonic Dystrophy

Myotonic dystrophy is a multisystem disorder transmitted by autosomal dominant inheritance (Adams, 2001). Symptoms usually begin in the second decade. An unstable DNA triplet in the DMPK gene (chromosome 19q13.2–13.3) causes the disease. Repeats may increase 50 to several thousand times in successive generations. The number of repeats correlates with the severity of disease, but repeat size alone does not predict phenotype. Repeat size changes from mother to child are greater than from father to child, and for this reason, the mother is usually the affected parent when a child has CMD. A mother with repeats of 100 units has a 90% chance that her child will have repeats of 400 units or more.

The main features during pregnancy are reduced fetal movement and polyhydramnios. Fifty percent of babies are born prematurely. Inadequate uterine contraction may prolong labor and forceps assistance is common. Severely affected newborns have inadequate diaphragmatic and intercostal muscle function and are incapable of spontaneous respiration. In the absence of prompt intubation and mechanical ventilation, many will die immediately after birth.

Prominent clinical features in the newborn include facial diplegia, in which the mouth is oddly shaped so that the upper lip forms an inverted V; generalized muscular hypotonia; joint deformities ranging from bilateral clubfoot to generalized arthrogryposis; and gastrointestinal dysfunction, including choking, regurgitation, aspiration, swallowing difficulties, and gastroparesis. Limb weakness in the newborn is more often proximal than distal. Tendon reflexes are usually absent in weak muscles. Percussion does not elicit myotonia in newborns, nor is EMG a reliable test.

Neonatal mortality is 16%, a frequent cause of death being cardiomyopathy. Survivors usually gain strength and are able to walk; however, a progressive myopathy similar to the late-onset form occurs eventually. Severe mental retardation is the rule, and may result from a combination of early respiratory failure and a direct effect of the mutation on the brain.

- **Diagnosis.** The diagnosis of congenital myotonic dystrophy in the newborn requires examination of the mother. She is likely to have many clinical features of the disease and show myotonia on EMG. Showing DNA amplification on chromosome 19 in both mother and child confirms the diagnosis. Test nonsymptomatic family members at risk for the carrier state.
- **Management.** The immediate treatment is intubation and mechanical ventilation. Fixed joints respond to physical therapy and casting. Metoclopramide alleviates gastroparesis.

METABOLIC MYOPATHIES

Acid Maltase Deficiency (Pompe Disease)

Acid maltase is a lysosomal enzyme, present in all tissues, that hydrolyzes maltose and other branches of glycogen to yield glucose. It has no function in maintaining blood glucose concentrations. Three distinct clinical forms of deficiency are recognized: infantile, childhood (see Ch. 7), and adult. Transmission of all forms is by autosomal recessive inheritance. The defective gene site is chromosome 17q25.2–25.3.

- **Clinical features.** The infantile form may begin immediately after birth but usually appears during the second month. Profound generalized hypotonia without atrophy and congestive heart failure are the initial symptoms. Hypotonia is the result of glycogen storage in the brain, spinal cord, and skeletal muscles, causing mixed signs of cerebral and motor unit dysfunction: decreased awareness and depressed tendon reflexes. The mixed signs may be confusing, but the presence of cardiomegaly is almost diagnostic. The electrocardiogram shows abnormalities, including short PR intervals and high QRS complexes on all leads. Most patients die of cardiac failure by 1 year of age.

  Characteristic of a second, milder subtype of the infantile form is less severe cardiomyopathy, absence of left ventricular outflow obstruction, and less than 5% of residual acid maltase activity. Longer survival is possible with assisted ventilation and intubation (Slonim et al., 2000).
- **Diagnosis.** Muscle biopsy establishes the diagnosis. Muscle fibers contain large vacuoles packed with glycogen. Acid maltase activity is deficient in fibroblasts and other tissues.
- **Management.** A phase I/II open-label single-dose study of recombinant human alpha-glucosidase infused intravenously twice weekly in 3 infants with infantile GSD II showed a steady decrease in heart size and maintenance of normal cardiac function for more than 1 year in all three infants (Amalfitano et al., 2001). Improvements of skeletal muscle functions also occurred.

Cytochrome-c-Oxidase Deficiency

The electron transfer chain and oxidative phosphorylation are the principal sources of adenosine triphosphate (ATP) synthesis (see Ch. 8). Deficiencies of mitochondrial enzymes that comprise the electron transfer chain in skeletal muscle may cause hypotonia in newborns or infants and exercise intolerance in older children. Deficiency of COX causes several different neuromuscular and cerebral disorders in childhood. Deficiency can result from mutations in either nuclear or mitochondrial DNA. Inheritance of most isolated COX deficiencies is autosomal recessive and caused by mutations in nuclear-encoded genes (Shoubridge, 2001). Most cases are sporadic.

- **Clinical features.** Clinical features vary with the number of enzyme deficiencies, the percentage reduction in enzyme activity, and the presence of mitochondrial enzyme deficiencies in organs other than muscle. Profound generalized weakness, causing difficulty in feeding, early respiratory failure, and death; severe lactic acidosis; and the De Toni–Fanconi–Debré syndrome (glycosuria, proteinuria, phosphaturia, and generalized aminoaciduria) characterize the complete syndrome. Onset is anytime within the first 6 months. Ptosis, ophthalmoplegia, and macroglossia may be present. Newborns with multiple enzyme deficiencies in multiple organs die within 6 months.
- **Diagnosis.** Suspect a deficiency in respiratory chain enzymes in any hypotonic infant with lactic acidosis. The serum concentration of CK is elevated, but EMG findings may be normal. Muscle biopsy reveals vacuoles, mainly in type I fibers, with abnormal glycogen and lipid accumulations. Mitochondria are large, increased in number, and abnormal in structure (ragged-red fibers).
- **Management.** No effective treatment is available for infants with overwhelming disease caused by multiorgan enzyme deficiency.

Myophosphorylase Deficiency

Enzyme deficiency results in an inability to metabolize glucose through fructose to lactate. Skeletal muscle is involved exclusively. The gene map locus is 11q13.

- **Clinical features.** The usual clinical syndrome of myophosphorylase deficiency (McArdle disease) is exercise intolerance in young adults. A rare neonatal form of variable severity exists whose mode of inheritance is autosomal recessive. One infant with severe McArdle disease developed progressive generalized weakness at age 4 weeks and died at age 13 weeks of respiratory failure. Muscle showed complete lack of phosphorylase activity. A premature infant of consanguineous parents showed joint contractures and clinical features of perinatal asphyxia.

  Affected newborns have difficulty with sucking and swallowing immediately postpartum or in the early neonatal period. In some, weakness is so profound that it produces immediate respiratory insufficiency. In others, weakness is progressive over several months or years. The child appears alert and has normal cranial nerve function. The tongue and heart are not affected. Tendon reflexes are depressed or absent.

- **Diagnosis.** The serum concentration of CK is elevated, and the EMG findings are abnormal, with features of both neuropathy and myopathy. Muscle biopsy is diagnostic. Fibers vary in size from atrophic to normal and contain peripheral vacuoles that react intensely for glycogen. The glycogen concentration of muscle is greatly elevated, and phosphorylase activity is undetectable.
- **Management.** Treatment is supportive.

RIGIDITY

Rigidity is very unusual in the newborn and most often encountered as part of tonic seizures, opisthotonic posturing, and decerebrate rigidity. Tetany from transitory hypocalcemia is the most common neuromuscular cause of rigidity (Table 3–8). Onset is usually during the second week postpartum, and the muscular rigidity is in response to stimulation.

Stiff Baby Syndrome

Other names for this syndrome are *hyperekplexia* and *Startle disease* (Scarcella and Coppola, 1997). The cause is a defect in the alpha-1 subunit of the glycine receptor, which maps to chromosome 5q32. Genetic transmission is either by autosomal dominant or recessive inheritance.

- **Clinical features.** The main clinical feature in the newborn is generalized stiffness that becomes worse on startle or handling. The trunk muscles may also be affected and respiration impaired. Tone is normal during sleep. Later in life, the main feature is generalized stiffness on startle.
- **Diagnosis.** Diagnosis is mainly clinical and the main use of laboratory tests is to exclude other pathological processes, especially myotonia.
- **Management.** Clonazepam provides partial relief from the stiffness. Other benzodiazepines, valproate, and levetiracetam may also be helpful.

TABLE 3–8   Stiffness (rigidity) in the newborn

Hyperekplexia
Tetany (hypocalcemia)
Tetanus (bacterial)
Neuromyotonia
Trilaminar myopathy

Schwartz–Jampel Syndrome

The Schwartz–Jampel syndrome (SJS) is a hereditary disorder, transmitted by autosomal recessive inheritance. The gene locus maps to 1p36.1. Characteristic features include short stature, skeletal abnormalities, and persistent muscular contraction and hypertrophy.

- **Clinical features.** Bone deformities are not prominent at birth. Continuous motor unit activity (CMUA) of the face is the main feature producing a characteristic triad that includes narrowing of the palpebral fissures (blepharophimosis), pursing of the mouth, and puckering of the chin. Striking or even blowing on the eyelids induces blepharospasm. CMUA in the limbs produces stiffness of gait and exercise intolerance. Motor development during the first year is slow, but intelligence is normal. A more severe neonatal form shows microcephaly with disproportion between skull and facial structures (Pinto-Escalante et al., 1997). Most die from respiratory complications in the first two years.
- **Diagnosis.** EMG shows CMUA. Initial reports suggested incorrectly that the abnormal activity seen on the EMG and expressed clinically was myotonia. Myotonia may be present, but CMUA is responsible for the facial and limb symptoms. The serum concentration of creatine kinase (CK) can be mildly elevated. The histological appearance of the muscle is usually normal but may show variation in fiber size and an increased number of central nuclei.
- **Management.** Phenytoin or carbamazepine diminishes the muscle stiffness. Early treatment with relief of muscle stiffness reduces the severity of subsequent muscle deformity.

REFERENCES AND FURTHER READING

Adams C. Myotonic dystrophy. (Updated 14 August 2001). In: GeneClinics: Medical Genetic Knowledge Base [database online] University of Washington. Available at http://www.geneclinics.org

Amalfitano A, Bengur AR, Morse RP, et al. Recombinant human acid alpha-glucosidase enzyme therapy for infantile glycogen storage disease type II: results of a phase I/II clinical trial. Genet Med 2001;3:132–138.

Axelrod FB, Goldberg JD, Ye XY, et al. Survival in familial dysautonomia: Impact of early intervention. J Pediatr 2002;141:518–523.

Cassidy SB and Schwartz S. Prader Willi syndrome. (Updated 8 April 2004). In: GeneClinics: Medical Genetic Knowledge Base [database online]. University of Washington. Available at http://www. geneclinics.org

Cherington M. Clinical spectrum of botulism. Muscle Nerve 1998;21:701–710.

Das S and Herman GD. X linked myotubular myopathy. (Updated 3 May 2004). In: GeneClinics: Medical Genetic Knowledge Base [database online]. University of Washington. Available at http://www. geneclinics.org

Escalante D, Ceballos-Quintal JM and Canto-Herrera J. Identical twins with the classical form of Schwartz–Jampel syndrome. Clin Dysmorph 1997;6:45–49.

Flanigan KM, Kerr L and Bromberg MB. Congenital muscular dystrophy with rigid spine syndrome. A clinical, pathological, radiological, and genetic study. Ann Neurol 2000;47:152–161.

Gordon E, Hoffman EP and Pegoraro E. Congenital muscular dystrophy overview. (Updated 2 January 2004). In: GeneClinics: Medical Genetic Knowledge Base [database online]. University of Washington. Available at http://www.geneclinics.org

Gordon E, Hoffman EP and Pegoraro E. Congenital muscular dystrophy overview. (Updated 25 March 2005). In: GeneClinics: Medical Genetic Knowledge Base [database online] University of Washington. Available at http://www.geneclinics.org

Grohmann K, Varon R, Stolz P, et al. Infantile spinal muscular atrophy with respiratory distress type 1 (SMARD). Ann Neurol 2003;54:719–724.

Harriette TFM, van der Zwaag B, Cruysberg JRM, et al. Mobius syndrome redefined. A syndrome of rhombencephalic maldevelopment. Neurology 2003;61:327–333.

Hoff JM, Daltveit AK and Gilhus NE. Myasthenia gravis. Consequences for pregnancy, delivery, and the newborn. Neurology 2003;61:1362–1366.

Ishikawa H, Sugie K, Murayama K, et al. Ullrich disease, Collagen VI deficiency. EM suggests a new basis for molecular weakness. Neurology 2002;59:920–923.

Jones KJ, Morgan G, Johnston H, et al. The expanding phenotype of laminin a$_2$ chain (merosin) abnormalities: Case series and review. J Med Genet 2001;38:649–657.

Lin T, Lewis RA and Nussbaum RL. Molecular confirmation of carriers for Lowe syndrome. Ophthalmology 1999;106:119–122.

Longman C, Brockington M, Torelli S, et al. Mutations in the human LARGE gene cause MDC1D, a novel form of congenital muscular dystrophy with severe mental retardation and abnormal glycosylation of alpha-dystroglycan. Hum Mol Genet 2003;12:2853–2861.

Miller SP, Riley P and Shevell MI. The neonatal presentation of Prader–Willi syndrome revisited. J Pediat 1999;134:226–228.

Monnier N, Romero NB, Lerale J, et al. An autosomal dominant congenital myopathy with cores and rods is associated with a neomutation in the RYR1 gene encoding the skeletal muscle ryanodine receptor. Hum Mol Genet 2000;9:2599–2608.

Mullaney P, Vajsar J, Smith R, et al. The natural history and ophthalmic involvement in childhood myasthenia gravis at The Hospital for Sick Children. Ophthalmology 2000;107:504–510.

North N. (Updated 25 November, 2002). Nemaline myopathy. In: GeneClinics: Medical Genetic Knowledge Base [database online]. University of Washington. Available at http://www.geneclinics.org

Philpot J, Cowan F, Pennock J, et al. Merosin-deficient muscular dystrophy: The spectrum of brain involvement on magnetic resonance imaging. Neuromusc Disord 1999;9:81–85.

Prior TW and Russman BS. (Updated 17 October, 2003). Spinal muscular atrophy. In: GeneClinics: Medical Genetic Knowledge Base [database online]. University of Washington. Available at http://www.geneclinics.org

Rees MI, Lewis TM, Kwok JBJ, et al. Hyperekplexia associated with compound heterozygote mutations in the beta-subunit of the human inhibitory glycine receptor (GLRB). Hum Mol Genet 2002;11:853–860.

Shohat M. (Updated 11 January, 2005). Familial dysautonomia. In: GeneClinics: Medical Genetic Knowledge Base [database online]. University of Washington. Available at http://www.geneclinics.org

Shoubridge EA. Cytochrome *c* oxidase deficiency. Am J Med Genet 2001;106:46–52.

Slonim AE, Bulone L, Ritz S, et al. Identification of two subtypes of infantile acid maltase deficiency. J Pediat 2000;137:283–285.

Steinberg SJ, Raymond GV, Braverman NE, et al. Peroxisome biogenesis disorders, Zellweger syndrome spectrum. (Updated 12 December 2003). In: GeneClinics: Medical Genetic Knowledge Base [database online]. University of Washington, Seattle. Available at http://www.geneclinics.org

Szigeti K, Saifi GM, Armstrong D, et al. Disturbance of muscle fiber differentiation in congenital hypomyelinating neuropathy caused by a novel myelin protein zero mutation. Ann Neurol 2003;54:398–402.

Wappner RS. Lowe Syndrome. (Updated 19 December 2003). In: GeneClinics: Medical Genetic Knowledge Base [database online]. University of Washington, Seattle. Available at http://www.geneclinics.org

4

Neonatal Hypoxic-Ischemic and Hemorrhagic Cerebral Injury

Elke H. Roland
and Alan Hill

Despite major advances in perinatal care, hypoxic-ischemic and hemorrhagic brain injuries are important causes of mortality and long-term neurological morbidity. Often, hypoxic-ischemic and hemorrhagic injury, in both premature and term newborns occur concomitantly, share many pathophysiological and etiological factors and have similar clinical features.

This chapter reviews the clinical aspects of neonatal hypoxic-ischemic and hemorrhagic brain injury and the current concepts of pathophysiology and neuropathology that have major clinical relevance.

HYPOXIC-ISCHEMIC BRAIN INJURY

A diagnosis of hypoxic-ischemic brain injury should be made cautiously, and only after detailed review of pregnancy, labor and delivery, other maternal risk factors, and family history. Epidemiological data demonstrates the importance of antepartum factors, often disregarded in earlier literature, in the genesis of chronic neurological disabilities in children. Only 12–20% of children with cerebral palsy and 10% of those with mental retardation relate directly to intrapartum hypoxic-ischemic insult (Nelson, 2003). Nevertheless, in absolute numbers, intrapartum injury still represents a significant cause of neurological morbidity and mortality.

The accurate diagnosis of antenatal hypoxic-ischemic brain injury may be problematic because infants who sustain injury earlier in gestation may be asymptomatic or exhibit few clinical abnormalities in the newborn period. In contrast, term newborns who sustain acute intrapartum hypoxic-ischemic insult of sufficient severity to result in long-term neurological sequelae are invariably encephalopathic during the newborn period. However, in some instances, such as newborns requiring sedation or complex life-support measures, the clinical features of the encephalopathy may be difficult to recognize. Another complicating issue is that the features of newborn encephalopathy are nonspecific and similar clinical features may be observable in the context of other brain insults, e.g. hemorrhage, infection, or metabolic. Thus, the importance of seeking evidence documenting the occurrence of a hypoxic-ischemic insult, e.g. prolonged fetal bradycardia or other abnormalities of fetal heart rate monitoring, low Apgar scores, low fetal scalp or cord pH, and requirement for prolonged resuscitation (Perlman, 1999). However, these clinical indicators of a prior hypoxic-ischemic insult do not necessarily predict brain injury or other adverse long-term outcomes.

Pathophysiology

Neonatal hypoxic-ischemic brain injury is associated with alterations in cerebral perfusion and cerebrovascular autoregulation as well as a cascade of metabolic derangements, e.g. decreased glucose substrates, lactic acidosis, accumulation of free radicals and toxic excitatory amino acids. Detailed discussion of these cellular and molecular mechanisms is outside the scope of this chapter.

The topography of hypoxic-ischemic cerebral injury is determined in large part by the stage of brain maturation at the time of insult and the severity and duration of injury. The maturity of the brain is a major determinant of the location of watershed zones of perfusion and of increased vulnerability of specific neuronal populations, e.g. neurons in brainstem nuclei, thalami and basal ganglia, which have a high metabolic rate in the newborn brain. For example, periventricular leukomalacia, a characteristic pattern of hypoxic-ischemic brain injury in the premature newborn, is determined principally by the location of vascular border zones of arterial perfusion in periventricular white matter and by selective vulnerability of oligodendrocyte precursors to hypoxic-ischemia (Volpe, 2001).

Experimental animal studies involving fetal primates have identified two major topographic patterns of injury that correlate with the temporal profile and severity of the intrapartum hypoxic-ischemic insult (Myers, 1975). Following 'acute total' hypoxia-ischemia of approximately 10–15 minutes duration, lesions were observed predominantly in brainstem nuclei and deep central gray matter structures, especially in the ventrolateral thalami and basal ganglia (putamen) with *relative* sparing of cortex and subcortical white matter. In contrast, the injury following less severe but prolonged asphyxia, occurring continuously or intermittently for longer than one hour, involves predominantly the cortex and subcortical white matter with *relative* preservation of central structures. In many instances, aspects of both types of injury occur with a predominance of one or the other type. Similar patterns of injury occur in the human term newborn (Roland et al., 1998; Pasternak and Gorey, 1998). However in the human newborn, an 'acute, total' insult (as was produced in the animal models) rarely, if ever, occurs, the closest approximation being cord prolapse, uterine rupture, massive placental abruption etc. In such instances, the insult should be more accurately termed as 'acute, near-total.'

Hypoxic-Ischemic Injury to Organs Other than Brain

Hypoxic-ischemic involvement of other organs, e.g. kidney, liver, heart, gastrointestinal system, provide supportive evidence of the occurrence of significant hypoxic-ischemia. However, it is difficult to establish the precise frequency of other organ involvement. Published studies vary widely in their definitions of asphyxia and in the criteria used to identify significant organ dysfunction (Martin-Ancel et al., 1995; Shah et al., 2004). In addition to the direct effects of hypoxic-ischemic injury, the redistribution of the fetal circulation that follows hypoxia-ischemia increases perfusion to vital organs (e.g. brain, heart, adrenal glands) and relatively decreases perfusion to other organs (diving reflex) exacerbating their injury.

In some instances, no evidence of systemic injury exists. This may occur following severe, acute, near-total asphyxia with abrupt and complete cessation of blood flow to the fetus. The redistribution of fetal circulation associated with the diving reflex may not occur and the brain may be the first organ to be injured (Jensen et al., 1999). Thus, several reports exist of newborns with hypoxic-ischemic encephalopathy (HIE) without significant multisystem involvement (Pasternak and Gorey, 1998; Phelan et al., 1998).

Clinical Encephalopathy

The occurrence of a clinically recognizable encephalopathy during the first days of life, preceded by evidence of intrapartum hypoxic-ischemic insult, is a *sine qua non* for the diagnosis of intrapartum hypoxic-ischemic encephalopathy (HIE). In premature newborns, the clinical features may be more difficult to recognize and best interpreted in the context of the gestational age of the infant (Volpe, 2005). Infants in whom intensive care procedures obscure the clinical features of encephalopathy are exceptions.

Although the onset of encephalopathy following hypoxic-ischemic insult ranges from 1–90 hours (Ahn et al., 1998), features of encephalopathy, such as seizures, usually occur during the first 24 hours. However, the diagnosis of neonatal seizures may be problematic (see Ch. 2). The clinical features may be subtle, e.g. limited to repetitive mouthing movements or eye deviation. In addition, clinical manifestations and electroencephalographic seizure activity on EEG may correlate poorly (Volpe, 2001).

Despite the wide spectrum of severity, HIE is often quantified for prognostic purposes as mild, moderate or severe (Miller et al., 2004; Robertson and Finer, 1993; Sarnat and Sarnat, 1976). Clinical features that distinguish between different grades of severity include level of consciousness, seizures, brainstem dysfunction including swallowing and feeding, and muscle tone (Table 4–1).

TABLE 4–1   Classification of severity of hypoxic-ischemic encephalopathy

Clinical features	Severity of encephalopathy		
	Mild	Moderate	Severe
Level of consciousness	Irritability	Drowsiness, lethargy	Coma
Seizures	Absent	Variable	Present
Tone	Normal or increased	Hypotonia	Severe hypotonia
Tendon reflexes	Increased	Variable	Decreased or absent
Primitive reflexes, e.g. Moro	Exaggerated	Decreased	Absent
Brainstem dysfunction including abnormal bulbar function	Absent	Variable	Present
Intracranial pressure (anterior fontanelle pressure)	Normal	Normal	Sometimes elevated
Outcome	Normal	Variable	Poor

Modified from Sarnat HB, Sarnat MS. Neonatal encephalopathy following fetal distress. Arch Neurol 1976;33: 696–705.

Severe Hypoxic Ischemic Encephalopathy

The term newborn generally has a predictable progression of abnormalities. Initial lethargy is often associated with preserved spontaneous respiratory function. After several hours, increased muscle tone and seizures are evident, followed by worsening hypotonia and unresponsiveness. The latter may be refractory to anticonvulsant therapy. In addition, signs of brainstem dysfunction occur (apnea, impaired eye movements, and bulbar dysfunction), which may culminate in respiratory arrest and death by 72 hours of age. Clinical evidence of cerebral edema, which may occur following a severe, prolonged-partial insult, often develops over the first 72 hours. Such edema implies extensive tissue necrosis. The use of anti-edema agents may decrease intracranial pressure, but does not improve outcome when cerebral perfusion is already maintained (Lupton et al., 1988). Cerebral edema, which may develop because of inappropriate secretion of antidiuretic hormone, requires careful monitoring of fluid balance.

Specific patterns of motor dysfunction that correlate with the topography of brain lesions are recognizable. For example, following injury to parasagittal watershed zones, hypotonia and weakness involve predominantly the shoulder girdle musculature. Infants with focal infarction may have unilateral weakness and premature newborns with injury to periventricular white matter often have abnormal tone affecting predominantly the legs. However, such patterns of motor abnormalities are often subtle and difficult to identify in the newborn infant.

Approximately 3 or 4 days following the original injury, seizures often abate, and the overall neurological status stabilizes. Improved alertness, hypotonia, and bulbar function may occur. However, following acute, near total HIE, brainstem dysfunction, e.g. facial diplegia, impaired sucking and swallowing, persist.

Topographical Patterns of Hypoxic-Ischemic Brain Injury

The various neuropathological patterns of neonatal hypoxic-ischemic injury are determined principally by the gestational age (maturity), the condition of the infant (e.g. small for gestational age, associated hypoglycemia) and the severity and duration of the hypoxic-ischemic insult (Table 4–2). The concomitant occurrence of other common adverse events, e.g. hypoglycemia, infection, and hemorrhage (discussed later) further complicates the relationship between the antecedent hypoxic-ischemic event and the subsequent brain injury. The patterns of injury differ significantly between term and premature newborns, and discussed separately.

Term Newborn

Cortical/Subcortical White Matter Injury (Including Parasagittal and Global Injury)
- **Pathogenesis.** Studies in experimental animals show a pattern of cortical and subcortical white matter injury occurs following approximately 60 minutes of partial hypoxic-ischemia. The insult may be continuous or intermittent. At the more severe end of the spectrum, extensive injury occurs

TABLE 4–2   Patterns of hypoxic-ischemic cerebral injury: correlation with gestational age and type of insult

Gestational age	Type of hypoxic-ischemic insult	Pattern of injury
Premature	Variable	Periventricular leukomalacia
	Variable	Periventricular hemorrhagic infarction
	Acute, near-total	Thalami > basal ganglia (putamen)
Term	Prolonged, partial	Cortex and subcortical white matter
		Parasagittal (watershed)
		Ulegyria (watershed)
		Global or diffuse
	Acute, near-total	Basal ganglia (esp. putamen) > thalami, brainstem nuclei
		± hippocampi
		± perirolandic cortex
		± white matter
	Combined prolonged, partial and acute, near-total	Combined pattern – unclassifiable
		Global or diffuse

to hemispheric structures with *relative* sparing of central gray matter, e.g. thalami, basal ganglia, brainstem. The most severe partial hypoxic-ischemic episode produces a global pattern of injury in which the entire brain is involved. Injuries following less severe partial hypoxic-ischemic episodes with a relatively minor reduction of overall cerebral perfusion, involve only the parasagittal cortex and subcortical white matter. These are the watershed zones of perfusion located between the territories supplied by the anterior, middle, and posterior cerebral arteries. Injury is usually bilateral, symmetrical, and more marked posteriorly.

- **Diagnosis.** Cerebral edema indicative of tissue necrosis is recognizable as increased echoes on cranial ultrasonography (US) or as low attenuation and decreased gray-white matter differentiation on computerized tomography (CT). Maximal edema occurs approximately 3 days following the hypoxic-ischemic event. However, the precise time of recognition of the decreased CT attenuation relates also to the severity of the injury. Magnetic resonance tomography (MRI) demonstrates these patterns of injury in greater detail (Fig. 4–1A,B). In the term newborn, conventional MRI (especially T2-weighted images) performed 8–10 days after the event most accurately demonstrates the extent of injury (Barnes, 2001). Diffusion-weighted MRI and magnetic resonance spectroscopy are more sensitive than conventional MRI for detection of injury in the early days of life. However, the results

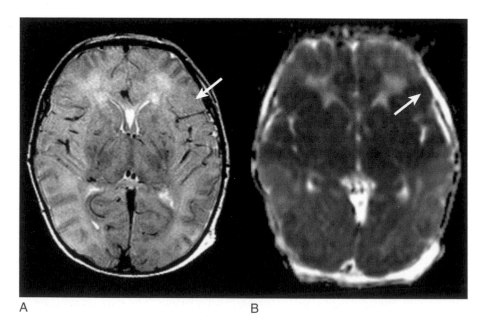

A   B

FIGURE 4–1   Axial T_2 weighted (A), and apparent diffusion coefficient (B) MR images of diffuse cortical, subcortical and central hypoxic-ischemic injury. Note loss of cortical ribbon on T_2 weighted MRI, which corresponds to region of restricted diffusion (arrows).

may be falsely negative or the magnitude of the lesions underestimated in scans obtained before 24 hours of age (Barkovich et al., 2001). The maximal decrease in diffusion coefficients are between 1–3 days following injury. After an acute injury, proton magnetic resonance imaging demonstrates a lactate peak in the first 24 hours followed by subsequent reduction in N-acetyl aspartate levels (Barkovich et al., 1999).

- **Clinical features.** Decreased level of consciousness, seizures, and hypotonia are the major clinical features of cortical injury. More restricted parasagittal injuries have hypotonia and weakness confined to the shoulder girdle musculature. These may be subtle and difficult to recognize. Seizures may be difficult to control during the first days of life. In severe cases, cerebral edema may be detectable clinically with bulging of the anterior fontanelle that appears maximal approximately 3 days after the insult. The condition of infants who survive beyond the first week stabilizes, but improvement may be limited. Long-term sequelae include cognitive impairment, cerebral palsy, and epilepsy. Specific deficits of language and visual-spatial perception may be a consequence of more posterior parasagittal injury (Erdogan, 2001).

Central Injury (Thalami, Basal Ganglia and Brainstem)

- **Pathogenesis.** As with cortical/subcortical white matter injury, initial documentation of the central injury pattern was in an experimental fetal primate model following acute, total asphyxia lasting approximately 10–20 minutes. In human newborns, this type of injury follows 'near-total' hypoxia-ischemia, and somewhat more prolonged episodes may be necessary to cause irreversible injury than was observed in the experimental animal studies. An important pathogenic factor is the high metabolic activity in the central gray matter structures of the newborn brain (e.g. extensive glutamatergic innervation of the basal ganglia) (Johnston et al., 2001). In addition, the areas of central injury are the watershed zones of the vertebrobasilar circulation in the fetal brainstem (Sarnat, 2004). At the more severe end of the spectrum of the acute, near-total insult, injury to hippocampi, perirolandic cortex and cerebellar vermis may occur (Sargent et al., 2004) (Figs 4–2A,B,C).
- **Diagnosis.** Although cranial ultrasonography may demonstrate increased echogenicity in deep, central structures, CT and especially MRI are superior for identification of injury to thalami and basal ganglia. MRI is required for recognition of injury to hippocampi, perirolandic cortex and cerebellum (Figs 4–3A,B,C). Documentation of brainstem injury remains difficult with all modalities, including conventional MRI (Sie et al., 2000 Miller et al., 2004).
- **Clinical features.** The hallmark of central injury is prominent and persistent brainstem dysfunction, e.g. requirement for prolonged ventilatory support, facial diplegia, gaze abnormalities, severely impaired sucking and swallowing and occasionally tongue fasciculations. The long-term sequelae generally include a mixed spastic and extrapyramidal cerebral palsy and persistent feeding difficulties that may lead to recurrent aspiration and require a gastrostomy feeding tube (Roland et al., 1998). The extrapyramidal component of the cerebral palsy may become evident only after several

years. Seizures may occur because of concomitant, albeit less severe cortical injury. Usually, head growth is relatively preserved, and few children
develop microcephaly (Mercuri et al., 2000).

Premature Infant

Premature newborns are at high risk for both hypoxic-ischemic and hemorrhagic brain injury, given the cardiorespiratory problems associated with

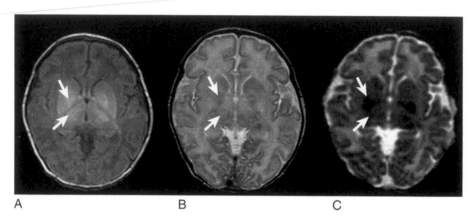

FIGURE 4–2   Axial T_1 (A) and T_2 (B) weighted, and apparent diffusion coefficient (C) MR images of central pattern of injury. Note bilateral involvement of ventrolateral nuclei of thalami and lentiform nuclei (arrows).

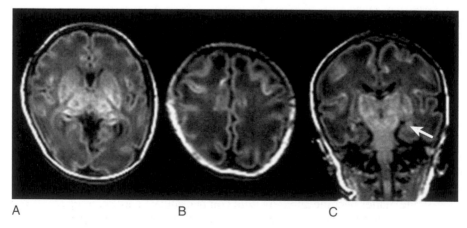

FIGURE 4–3   Axial T_1 (A, B), and coronal T_1 (C) weighted MR images of a central pattern of injury, following an acute near-total hypoxic-ischemic insult. Note T_1 shortening in thalami, basal ganglia and depths of sulci as well as bilateral hippocampal involvement (arrow showing lesion in left hippocampus).

prematurity, e.g. respiratory distress syndrome and pneumothorax, patent ductus arteriosus and apnea. In addition, premature newborns experience fluctuations in systemic blood pressure, often associated with routine caretaking maneuvers, which, in turn, result in a decrease of cerebral perfusion because of the pressure-passive cerebral circulation and impaired cerebrovascular autoregulation in the sick premature newborn. Clearly, with impaired cerebrovascular autoregulation, increases in systemic blood pressure and cerebral blood flow may result in rupture of the fragile vessels of the germinal matrix and hemorrhagic injury, whereas systemic hypotension may result in decreased cerebral perfusion and hypoxic-ischemic injury. Studies in preterm lambs have demonstrated that early in the process of maturation of cerebrovascular autoregulation, the range of blood pressures over which cerebral blood flow remains constant is narrow and even normal blood pressures are near the limits of the autoregulatory curve. Consequently, even healthy, stable premature infants with intact cerebrovascular autoregulation may be vulnerable to fluctuations in systemic blood pressure.

Periventricular Leukomalacia

- **Pathogenesis.** In premature newborns, hypoxic-ischemic injury has a predilection for the periventricular white matter, a border zone of arterial perfusion located between the ventriculofugal choroidal arteries and the ventriculopedal penetrating branches of the anterior, middle, and posterior cerebral arteries. The most vulnerable locations for such injury include the posterior white matter at the trigones of the lateral ventricles and the anterior white matter around the foramen of Monro and at the angles of the anterior horns of the lateral ventricles. The rich interarterial anastomoses of terminal branches of the anterior, middle, and posterior cerebral arteries in the premature brain relatively spares the cortex. However, more recently, neuropathological and volumetric MRI studies demonstrate a volume reduction of the cortex in association with periventricular leukomalacia (Inder et al., 1999; Pierson et al., 2003; Volpe, 2005).

  Beyond the vascular anatomical factors, an intrinsic vulnerability of differentiating oligodendrocytes to necrosis and subsequent apoptosis increases the vulnerability of the immature brain to diffuse white matter injury (Back et al., 2002). Experimental animal studies and human placental pathology indicate that inflammatory mediators (endotoxins and cytokines) may have a pathogenic role, although the precise mechanisms by which this occurs is not understood fully (Kadhim et al., 2003; Yoon et al., 2003).

- **Diagnosis.** Serial cranial ultrasound scans may identify severe periventricular leukomalacia based on increased, albeit transitory, echoes in periventricular white matter usually followed, after approximately 3–6 weeks, by cystic degeneration. After 2–3 months, collapse of the cysts and atrophy of white matter become apparent with compensatory ventriculomegaly. These produce a characteristic irregular appearance with scalloping of the ventricular walls. In some instances, the early increased echogenicity resolves without subsequent cyst formation.

  Despite mounting evidence that diffusion-weighted MRI may identify periventricular leukomalacia (PVL) in the early days of life (Counsell et al.,

2003), the role of CT and MRI for the early diagnosis of periventricular leu-komalacia has not been defined in detail. However, MRI may demonstrate small foci of white matter abnormalities not visualized by ultrasonography (Miller et al., 2002, 2003).

The late stages of PVL may appear on cranial ultrasonography as ven-triculomegaly with irregular outline of the ventricular walls (hydrocephalus ex vacuo). On CT, deep sulci may be observed, which, in severe cases abut almost directly on to the ventricular walls due to loss of the interposed white matter. However, MRI is now considered the imaging technique of choice for detection of late PVL in that it has the capability to demonstrate more extensive and diffuse signal changes in white matter that are not detected by ultrasonography or CT (Ment et al., 2002) (Figs 4–4A,B,C,D).

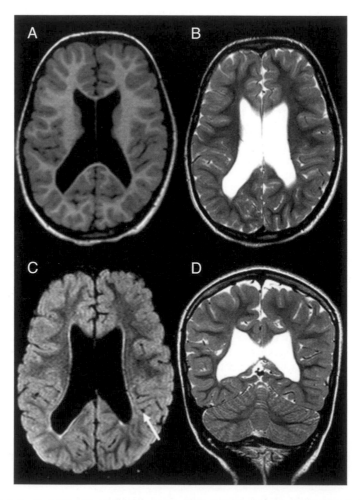

FIGURE 4–4   Axial T_1 (A) and T_2 (B) weighted, FLAIR (C), and coronal T_2 (D) MR images of endstage periventricular leukomalacia. Note ventriculomegaly with irregular ventricular border, loss of periventricular white matter and depths of sulci abutting the ventricular margin (arrow).

- **Clinical features.** During the newborn period, PVL may be associated with subtle abnormalities of tone and power in the legs. However, the recognition of such abnormalities may be difficult in the presence of complex life-support apparatus and other confounding types of injury, e.g. intraventricular hemorrhage. Spastic diplegia is the long-term sequelae of PVL. In more severe cases, spastic quadriplegia occurs with the legs more severely involved that the arms. This pattern of motor abnormality reflects the anatomical organization of motor fibers, where fibers subserving lower limb function descend most medially and are closest in proximity to the most common and severe regions of injury. Injury to the optic radiations results in visual impairment. Behavioral disturbances and intellectual deficits are associated with more diffuse or scattered foci of white matter injury (Volpe, 2005). Epilepsy occurs in almost half of patients with cerebral palsy and PVL diagnosed on MRI (Gurses and Gross, 1999). The white matter lesions interfere with the migration of subplate neurons from their origin in the subplate marginal zone to the cortex. This in turn, results in aberrant cortical synaptic connections, which may also contribute to the high incidence of associated cognitive and behavioral dysfunction (Volpe, 2005).

Periventricular Hemorrhagic Infarction
- **Pathogenesis.** Periventricular hemorrhagic infarction is unilateral or strikingly asymmetric hemorrhagic necrosis in the periventricular white matter located just dorsal and lateral to the external angles of the lateral ventricles. Although approximately 80% of cases are associated with large germinal matrix-intraventricular hemorrhage (GMH-IVH), PHI is not simply an 'extension' of the GMH-IVH, but rather represents a venous infarction resulting from obstruction of blood flow in the terminal vein by a large, ipsilateral germinal matrix hemorrhage (Counsell et al., 1999; de Vries et al., 2001). The incidence of periventricular hemorrhagic infarction correlates closely with gestational age, i.e. approximately one third occurs in infants of birth weight <700 g. Clearly, because the GMH plays such a major role in the pathogenesis of periventricular hemorrhagic infarction, the major risk factors identified for GMH-IVH are also relevant for periventricular hemorrhagic infarction (Gleissner et al., 2000; Linder et al., 2003). The unilateral lesion is distinguishable from periventricular leukomalacia, which represents arterial infarction and is typically bilateral. However, in many instances, both types of injury occur together and play a contributory role in the severity of neurological sequelae.
- **Diagnosis.** Visualization of periventricular hemorrhagic infarction is by cranial US, CT or MRI. Its appearance is a unilateral or asymmetric wedge- or fan-shaped hemorrhagic lesion in the periventricular white matter associated with large ipsilateral GMH-IVH (Counsell et al., 1999; de Vries et al., 2001) (Fig. 4–5).
- **Clinical features.** Clinical features include hemiparesis with more marked involvement of the legs, in contrast to the pattern of weakness following middle cerebral artery infarction that affects predominantly the arms. MRI evidence of direct injury or subsequent asymmetrical myelination of the posterior limb of the internal capsule at term predicts subsequent hemiplegia (de Vries et al., 2001). Cognitive impairment and epilepsy are a consequence

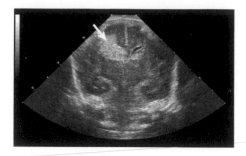

FIGURE 4–5   Cranial ultrasound (coronal view) of a right periventricular hemorrhagic infarction (arrow) and asymmetric intraventricular hemorrhage.

of concomitant cortical injury. Given that this lesion is usually associated with severe germinal matrix-intraventricular hemorrhage, affected infants are also at risk for the development of post-hemorrhagic hydrocephalus.

Management of hypoxic-ischemic encephalopathy

In most term newborns with acute HIE, the injury occurs primarily during labor and delivery. Hence, prevention depends on early recognition of maternal risk factors and close surveillance of the high-risk fetus during pregnancy, labor, and delivery. This topic falls primarily within the realm of obstetrics. Similarly, the management of dysfunction of systemic organs, albeit important, falls outside the scope of this chapter, which is limited to a discussion of the management of hypoxic-ischemic brain injury.

Maintenance of Adequate Ventilation and Perfusion

Although the principal hypoxic-ischemic insult often occurs before delivery, aggressive resuscitation and ongoing cardiorespiratory support are essential for the prevention of ongoing, hypoxic-ischemic injury. The practice of ventilation with oxygen, a routine part of acute resuscitation, is undergoing review. Concerns for the potential toxicity of oxygen include acute lung injury, bronchopulmonary dysplasia, and retinopathy of prematurity (Niermeyer et al., 2004). Furthermore, recent data suggest that the severity of newborn encephalopathy following resuscitation with room air may be no worse than that seen after resuscitation with 100% oxygen. This may reflect a reduction in the formation of oxygen free radicals when room air is used (Vento et al., 2002). However, significant changes in routine resuscitation procedures require long-term outcome comparison studies (Saugstad et al., 2003, 2004).

The presence of impaired cerebrovascular autoregulation in premature newborns and in critically ill term newborns, adds urgency to the rapid restoration of adequate cardiac output and the maintenance of normal systemic blood pressure. On the other hand, it is equally important to avoid systemic hypertension, which may increase the risk for intracranial hemorrhage. These aspects are especially important in premature infants in whom fluctuations in blood pressure (and hence cerebral perfusion) occur postnatally in association with routine handling, apnea, and patent ductus arteriosus with possible steal from the cerebral circulation. Another important consideration is the potential risks associated with hypocapnia or hypercapnia. Hypocapnea is associated with vigorous hyperventilation and may reduce cerebral perfusion. Conversely, normal or moderate hypercapnea may be neuroprotective with preservation of cerebral blood flow, oxidative phosphorylation, and lower cerebrospinal fluid levels of glutamate (Vannucci et al., 1995). The effects of newer ventilation techniques (e.g. high frequency ventilation, nitric oxide) on the cerebral circulation and injury have not been completely determined.

Maintenance of Metabolic Homeostasis

Several metabolic derangements, which have deleterious effects, may occur in the context of hypoxic-ischemic encephalopathy. The principal ones are lactic acidosis, hypoglycemia, and other electrolyte disturbances, e.g. hypocalcemia, hypomagnesemia, and hyponatremia. Experimental studies show that hypoglycemia may be associated with a two to three-fold increase in cerebral blood flow, which, in turn, may lead to increased risk for hemorrhagic injury (Chui et al., 1998). In addition, a synergistic detrimental relationship may exist between hypoglycemia and hypoxia-ischemia (Stevenson et al., 2003). Infants at increased risk for hypoglycemia include infants with reduced hepatic glycogen stores, such as preterm infants or growth-retarded newborns, infants with impaired glucose metabolism, e.g. infants of diabetic mothers, and infants with increased glucose consumption, e.g. hypothermia, hyperthermia or infection.

Control of Seizures

Seizures, a major feature of moderate or severe HIE, have several secondary effects, e.g. impairment of ventilation, increase in blood pressure, reduction of cerebral glucose and high-energy phosphate substrates, and accumulation of toxic excitatory amino acids. Evidence from experimental animal studies indicates an additional injurious effect of seizures on hypoxic-ischemic brain injury, which supports an aggressive approach to the treatment of seizures in the context of HIE (Wirrell et al., 2001). However, seizures may be refractory to treatment during the first days despite aggressive use of anticonvulsants. Clearly, following the correction of metabolic derangements that may contribute to seizure activity, such as hypoglycemia and hypocalcemia, treatment with anticonvulsant medications is required. Efficacy studies of anticonvulsants for treatment of neonatal seizures show that phenobarbital and phenytoin are equally effective when administered intravenously. Seizure control is less than 50% when using either drug alone, but increases to more than 60% with combined therapy (Painter et al., 1999, 2001). Fosphenytoin, a phosphorylated prodrug of phenytoin, has gained attention because it has fewer cardiovascular and cutaneous side effects. However, the conversion rate of fosphenytoin to phenytoin in young infants is uncertain, which necessitates individualization of dosage (Kriel et al., 2001). In refractory cases, benzodiazepines, e.g. intermittent doses of lorazepam or continuous midazolam infusion may be helpful.

The optimum duration of maintenance antiepileptic therapy varies from child to child, balancing the likelihood of seizure recurrence against the potentially deleterious effects of anticonvulsant drugs. Whenever possible, aim for a brief duration of treatment. The severity of the neonatal encephalopathy and the persistence of neurological and EEG abnormalities are important factors that may assist decisions concerning the duration of treatment.

Control of Brain Swelling

A bulging anterior fontanelle clinically indicates cerebral edema. Neuroimaging confirms the diagnosis. There is no evidence that antiedema agents (e.g. mannitol), improve ultimate neurological outcome when cerebral perfusion is already adequate.

Neuroprotective Strategies

Recent studies in experimental animals and human newborns have shown a biphasic pattern of cerebral energy failure following hypoxic-ischemic insult. The secondary phase of energy failure, which relates in part to mitochondrial dysfunction, occurs after a latent period of up to 24 hours. This may provide a window of opportunity for neuroprotective interventions. Although several interventions currently under investigation show encouraging results in animal models, (calcium channel blockers, allopurinol, oxypurinol), the most promising approach involves either whole body or selective head cooling. Thus, trials in human newborns with neonatal encephalopathy appear to show safety and dose-related improvements in mortality and long-term morbidity (Gluckman et al., 2005; Inder et al., 2004; Shankaran et al., 2004). Although the optimal timing and depth of hypothermia for neuroprotection in human infants are not established, brief, mild to moderate hypothermia of less than 3 hours' duration immediately following the hypoxic-ischemic episode has only modest, inconsistent effects whereas prolonged cooling for up to 72 hours appears to have greater benefit (Compagnoni et al., 2002). In addition to any direct benefit from cerebral cooling, this strategy may widen the window of opportunity for neuronal rescue by other therapeutic interventions (Shankaran, 2002).

GERMINAL MATRIX-INTRAVENTRICULAR HEMORRHAGE

The incidence of germinal matrix-intraventricular hemorrhage, which occurs principally in premature newborns, has declined in recent decades to less than

20%. It originates from rupture of fragile vessels in the subependymal germinal matrix. Serial neuroimaging shows that 50% originate during the first day and 90% occur before the fourth day. The hemorrhage enlarges during the first week in 20–40% of cases. The most common complications are posthemorrhagic hydrocephalus and periventricular hemorrhagic infarction (discussed earlier) (Sheth, 1998).

Pathogenesis

The pathogenesis of germinal matrix-intraventricular hemorrhage is multifactorial and involves intravascular, vascular, and extravascular factors (Table 4–3) (Linder et al., 2003; Roland and Hill, 2003). Intravascular factors involve the regulation of blood flow within the fragile vasculature of the germinal matrix, platelet-capillary interactions and coagulation disturbances. Vascular factors include the fragility of vessels in the germinal matrix and extravascular factors relate to the characteristics of the supporting tissues. In many instances, concomitant or antecedent hypoxic-ischemic insult contributes to brain injury.

Acute ventricular enlargement may occur in the context of massive GMH-IVH. More commonly, progressive ventriculomegaly develops gradually over several weeks because of impaired cerebrospinal fluid reabsorption secondary to obliterative arachnoiditis in the posterior fossa, impairment of CSF outflow at the aqueduct by clot or CSF resorption from blockage of small arachnoid villi by particulate debris. Often there is a delay in the clinical manifestation of increased intracranial pressure due to the generous subarachnoid spaces in the immature brain and the high compliance of the periventricular tissue, especially in the context of prior hypoxic-ischemic insult.

Intraventricular hemorrhage occurs also in a small percentage of term newborns, often in association with hypoxic-ischemic or traumatic injury. The sites of origin of IVH in term newborns are more variable and include residual germinal matrix, choroid plexus, vascular malformation, or venous infarction of the

TABLE 4–3 Major risk factors for germinal matrix-intraventricular hemorrhage

Pathogenic factors	*Risk factors*
Alterations in cerebral blood flow	Immature cerebrovascular autoregulation
	Mechanical ventilation
	Hypoxic-ischemic insult
	Anemia
	Hypoglycemia
Increase in cerebral venous pressure	Labor
	Vaginal delivery
	Respiratory distress syndrome
Coagulation disturbances	Disseminated intravascular coagulation
Fragility of germinal matrix vessels	Hypoxic-ischemic insult
	Chorioamnionitis, sepsis
Deficient vascular support of germinal matrix	Dehydration, low blood volume

thalamus. The latter entity often presents later at several days or weeks of age (Roland et al., 1990).

- **Diagnosis.** Cranial ultrasonography (US) is the neuroimaging modality of choice for diagnosis of GMH-IVH. US is indicated at least once between 7 and 14 days of age in all infants less than 30 weeks' gestation and earlier if there are specific concerns. Subsequent serial scans every 1 to 2 weeks, as indicated, monitor ventricular size and possible development of posthemorrhagic hydrocephalus. Computed tomography or MRI may be required to differentiate between ischemic and hemorrhagic lesions (Ment et al., 2002).

  Classification of the severity of GMH-IVH on US follows:

  Grade 1: Isolated germinal matrix hemorrhage

  Grade 2: Intraventricular hemorrhage without ventricular dilatation

  Grade 3: Intraventricular hemorrhage with ventricular dilatation

  Grade 4: Intraventricular and parenchymal hemorrhage with ventricular dilatation.

While this grading system has some correlation with prognosis, the prognosis with 'Grade 4' GMH-IVH relates more to the location and extent of parenchymal involvement.

Clinical Features

Clinical features alone suggest the diagnosis of GMH-IVH in only half of cases (Volpe, 2001). The spectrum of severity of clinical abnormalities ranges from an asymptomatic state through saltatory neurological deterioration over several days to catastrophic deterioration resulting in coma, apnea, extensor posturing, and brainstem dysfunction. Associated systemic abnormalities include hypotension, metabolic acidosis, and bradycardia.

A delay in the clinical signs of posthemorrhagic hydrocephalus, e.g. excessively rapid head growth, bulging anterior fontanelle, and suture diastasis, may be days or weeks after serial ultrasound scans indicate the onset of progressive ventricular dilation.

Management

The optimal management strategy for prevention of GMH-IVH is by prevention of premature labor and delivery. However, even temporary delay of premature delivery for several days may permit the administration of antenatal corticosteroids. Corticosteroids induce the maturation of fetal lungs, thereby reducing postnatal respiratory distress syndrome and cardiorespiratory disturbances that contribute to GMH-IVH, and the maturation of fragile vessels within the germinal matrix (Crowley, 2000). As discussed in the earlier section on HIE, the prevention or correction of hemodynamic disturbances and the maintenance of adequate ventilation may reduce the overall incidence and severity of GMH-IVH. Although abnormal coagulation may play a role in the causation of

GMH-IVH, combined data from randomized trials to date have failed to demonstrate a reduction of severe GMH-IVH or mortality with routine use of volume expansion, with saline, plasma, albumin, or blood substitutes. Indomethacin, used for treatment of symptomatic patent ductus arteriosus, may be associated with lower incidence of severe GMH-IVH without apparent adverse long-term effects (Fowlie and Davis, 2002).

Progressive ventriculomegaly occurs in approximately 25–35% of infants with GMH-IVH and may resolve spontaneously (either totally or partially) usually within four weeks of onset (Fig. 4–6). Recent data suggests that the natural history of posthemorrhagic hydrocephalus may be evolving such that a greater percentage, i.e. approximately two-thirds of affected infants, requires active intervention (Murphy et al., 2002). Complicating the decision concerning timing of intervention is that the clinical criteria for diagnosing the deleterious

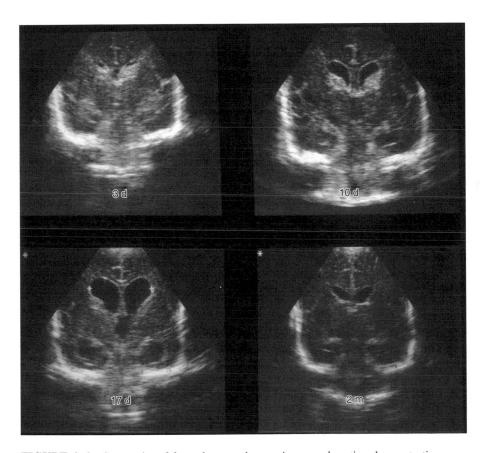

FIGURE 4–6 Composite of four ultrasound scans in coronal section demonstrating ventriculomegaly after intraventricular hemorrhage at 3 days of age, with spontaneous resolution by 2 months of age.

effects of increased intracranial pressure lack sensitivity and are often delayed (du Plessis, 1998). Although serial ultrasound scans may identify progressive dilatation prior to the development of clinical abnormalities, standardized measurements of ventricular size are nonexistent. Useful observations suggestive of progressive hydrocephalus include rapidly progressively ventriculomegaly, prominent dilatation of temporal horns of the lateral ventricles, a hyperechoic outline in periventricular regions and decrease in ventricular size following removal of cerebrospinal fluid.

No reduction in mortality, severity of neurological sequelae, or requirement for permanent shunt replacement follows early 'prophylactic' interventions such as cerebrospinal fluid drainage (Whitelaw, 2000) or intraventricular fibrinolytic therapy (Whitelaw, 2001) prior to the development of progressive ventriculomegaly. Similarly, drug therapy e.g. acetazolamide, furosemide, osmotic agents, is neither safe nor effective (Whitelaw et al., 2001). Temporizing interventions during the first weeks of life prior to permanent shunt placement include CSF drainage by serial lumbar punctures, external ventricular drainage, and the use of a subcutaneous ventricular access device or ventriculosubgaleal shunt. These procedures may be effective if it is technically feasible to remove sufficient fluid (i.e. 10–15 mL/kg/day for a minimum of 2–3 weeks). Definitive treatment involves permanent ventricular drainage by shunt placement into the peritoneal cavity or venous system. The optimal timing for permanent shunt placement remains controversial. Recent studies show no correlation between timing of shunt placement and outcome (Resch et al., 1996; Taylor and Peter, 2001).

The major obstacle to developing a rational strategy for the management of germinal matrix-intraventricular hemorrhage and posthemorrhagic ventriculomegaly is the inability to diagnose precisely the extent and onset of associated hypoxic-ischemic and other brain injury in the premature newborns in whom there are multiple concomitant mechanisms of injury.

Outcome

The outcome for premature newborns with GMH-IVH relates to the severity of the hemorrhage, complications of posthemorrhagic hydrocephalus and periventricular hemorrhagic infarction and concomitant hypoxic-ischemic injury, e.g. periventricular leukomalacia. The latter appears to be the most critical determinant of outcome. Infants with small GMH-IVH alone often have no major sequelae whereas the incidence of major sequelae increases to 30–40% following severe hemorrhage. The extent and location of parenchymal involvement is the principal determinant for prediction of outcome. Thus, localized parenchymal involvement confined to frontal, or occipital regions has more favorable outcome. The risk for major sequelae is also high in infants with posthemorrhagic hydrocephalus, especially in those who require a ventriculoperitoneal shunt. Multicenter studies report a morbidity rate between 20–35% and moderate or severe impairment in 50–75% of survivors (Resch et al., 1996; Hamigan et al., 1991).

REFERENCES AND FURTHER READING

Ahn MO, Korst LM, Phelan JP, et al. Does the onset of neonatal seizures correlate with the timing of fetal neurologic injury? Clin Pediatr 1998;37:673–676.

Back SA, Han PH, Luo NL, et al. Selective vulnerability of late oligodendrocyte progenitors to hypoxia-ischemia. J Neurosci 2002;22:455–446.

Barkovich AJ, Baranski K, Vigneron D, et al. Proton MR spectroscopy for the evaluation of brain injury in asphyxiated, term neonates. Am J Neuroradiol 1999;20:1399–1405.

Barkovich AJ, Westmark KD, Bedi HS, et al. Proton spectroscopy and diffusion imaging on the first day of life after perinatal asphyxia: Preliminary report. Am J Neuroradiol 2001;22:1786–1794.

Barnes PD. Neuroimaging and the timing of fetal and neonatal brain injury. J Perinatol 2001;21:44–66.

Chiu NT, Huang CC, Chang YC, et al. Technetium-99m-HMPAO brain SPECT in neonates with hypoglycemic encephalopathy. J Nucl Med 1998;39:1711–1713.

Compagnoni G, Pogliani L, Lista G, et al. Hypothermia reduces neurological damage in asphyxiated newborn infants. Biol Neonate 2002;82:222.

Counsell SJ, Allsop JM, Harrison MC, et al. Diffusion-weighted imaging of the brain in preterm infants with focal and diffuse white matter abnormality. Pediatrics 2003;112:1–7.

Counsell SJ, Maalouf ER, Rutherford MA, et al. Periventricular haemorrhagic infarct in a preterm neonate. Eur J Paediatr Neurol 1999;3:25–28.

Crowley P. Prophylactic cortico steroids for preterm birth. Cochrane Database Syst Rev 2:CD 000065; 2000.

de Vries LS, Roelants-van Rijn AM, Rademaker KJ, et al. Unilateral parenchymal haemorrhagic infarction in the preterm infant. Eur J Paediatr Neurol 2001;5:139–149.

Du Plessis AJ. Posthemorrhagic hydrocephalus and brain injury in the preterm infant: dilemmas in diagnosis and management. Semin Pediat Neurol 1998;5:161–179.

Erdogan N. Parasagittal injury in infants with hypoxic-ischemic encephalopathy. J Child Neurol 2001;6:299–300.

Fowlie PW and Davis PG. Prophylactic intravenous Indomethacin for preventing mortality and morbidity in preterm infants. Cochrane Database Syst. Rev 3: CD000174; 2002.

Gleissner M, Jorch G and Avenarius S. Risk factors for intraventricular hemorrhage in a birth cohort of 3721 premature infants. J Perinat Med 2000;28:104–110.

Gluckman PD, Wyatt JS, Azzopardi D, et al. Selective head cooling with mild systemic hypothermia after neonatal encephalopathy: Multicenter randomized trial. Lancet 2005;365:663.

Gurses C, Gross DW, Andermann F, et al. Periventricular leukomalacia and epilepsy: incidence and seizure pattern. Neurology 1999;52:341–345.

Hamigan W, Morgan A, Anderson R, et al. Incidence and neurodevelopmental outcome of periventricular hemorrhage and hydrocephalus in a regional population of very low birthweight infants. Neurosurgery 1991;29:701–706.

Inder TE, Hunt RW, Morley CJ, et al. Randomized trial of systemic hypothermia selectively protects the cortex on MRI in term hypoxic-ischemic encephalopathy. J Pediatrics 2004;145:835.

Inder TE, Huppi PS, Warfield S, et al. Periventricular white matter injury in the premature infant is followed by reduced cerebral cortical gray matter volume at term. Ann Neurol 1999;46:755–760.

Jensen A, Garmier Y and Berger R. Dynamics of fetal circulatory responses to hypoxia and asphyxia. Eur J Obstet Gynecol Reprod Biol 1999;84:155–172.

Johnston MV, Trescher WH, Ishada A, et al. Neurobiology of hypoxic-ischemic injury in the developing brain. Pediatr Res 2001;49:735–741.

Kadhim H, Tabarki B, de Prez C, et al. Cytokine immunoreactivity in cortical and subcortical neurons in periventricular leukomalacia: are cytokines implicated in neuronal dysfunction in cerebral palsy? Acta Neuropathol 2003;105:209–216.

Kriel RL and Cifuentes RF. Fosphenytoin in infants of extremely low birth weight. Pediatr Neurol 2001;24:219–221.

Linder N, Haskin O, Levit O, et al. Risk factors for intraventricular hemorrhage in very low birth weight premature infants: a retrospective case-control study. Pediatrics 2003;111:590–595.

Lupton BA, Hill A, Roland EH, et al. Brain swelling in the asphyxiated term newborn: pathogenesis and outcome. Pediatrics 1988;82:129–146.

Martin-Ancel A, Garcia-Alix A, Gaya F, et al. Multiple organ involvement in perinatal asphyxia. J Pediatr 1995;127:786–793.

Ment LR, Bada HS, Barnes P, et al. Practice parameter: neuroimaging of the neonate. Neurology 2002;58:1726–1738.

Mercuri E, Ricci D, Cowan RM, et al. Head growth in infants with hypoxic-ischemic encephalopathy: correlation with neonatal magnetic resonance imaging. Pediatrics 2000;106:235–243.

Miller SP, Cozzio CC, Goldstein RB, et al. Comparing the diagnosis of white matter injury in premature newborns with serial MR imaging and transfontanel ultrasonography findings. Am J Neuroradiol 2003;24:1661–1669.

Miller SP, Latal B, Clark H, et al. Clinical signs predict 30-month neurodevelopmental outcome after neonatal encephalopathy. Am J Obstet Gynecol 2004;190:93–99.

Miller SP, Ramaswamy V, Michelson D, et al. Patterns of brain injury in term neonatal encephalopathy. J Pediatr 2005;146:453–460.

Miller SP, Vigneron DB, Henry RG, et al. Serial quantitative diffusion tensor MRI of the premature brain: development in newborns with and without injury. J Magn Reson Imaging 2002;16:621–632.

Murphy BP, Inder TE, Rooks V, et al. Posthemorrhagic ventricular dilatation in the premature infant: natural history and predictors of outcome. Arch Dis Child Fetal Neonatal Ed 2002;87:F37–41.

Myers RE. Four patterns of perinatal brain damage and their condition of occurrence in primates. In: BS Meldrum and CD Marsden, eds. Advances in Neurology, Vol. 10, New York: Raven Press, 1975.

Nelson KB. Can we prevent cerebral palsy? N Engl J Med. 2003;349:1765–1769.

Niermeyer S and Vento M. Is 100% oxygen necessary for the resuscitation of newborn infants? J Matern Fetal Neonatal Med 2004;15:75–84.

Painter MJ and Alvin J. Neonatal seizures. Curr Treat Options Neurol 2001;3:237–248.

Painter MJ, Scher MS, Stein AD, et al. Phenobarbital compared with phenytoin for the treatment of neonatal seizures. N Engl J Med 1999;341:485–489.

Pasternak JF, Gorey MT. The syndrome of near-total intrauterine asphyxia in the term infant. Pediatr Neurol 1998;18: 391–398.

Perlman JM. Markers of asphyxia and neonatal brain injury. N Engl J Med 1999;341:328–335.

Phelan JP, Ahn MO, Korst L, et al. Intrapartum fetal asphyxial brain injury with absent multiorgan system dysfunction. J Matern Fetal Med 1998;7:19–22.

Pierson CR, Folkerth RD, Haynes RL, et al. Gray matter injury in premature infants with or without periventricular leukomalacia (PVL). J Neuropathol Exp Neurol 2003;62:518.

Resch B, Gedermann A, Maurer U, et al. Neurodevelopmental outcome of hydrocephalus following intra/periventricular hemorrhage in preterm infants: short and longterm results. Child's Nerv Syst 1996;12:27–33.

Robertson CMT, Finer NN. Long-term follow-up of term neonates with perinatal asphyxia. Clin Perinatol 1993;20:483–500.

Roland EH, Flodmark O, Hill A. Thalamic hemorrhage with intraventricular hemorrhage in the full-term newborn. Pediatrics 1990;85:737–742.

Roland EH, Hill A. Germinal matrix-intraventricular hemorrhage in the premature newborn: Management and outcome. Neurol Clin 2003;21:833–851.

Roland EH, Poskitt K, Rodriguez E, et al. Perinatal hypoxic-ischemic thalamic injury: Clinical features and neuroimaging. Ann Neurol 1998;44:161–166.

Sargent MA, Poskitt KJ, Roland EH, et al. Cerebellar vermian atrophy after neonatal hypoxic-ischemic encephalopathy. Am J Neuroradiol 2004;25:1008–1015.

Sarnat HB, Sarnat MS. Neonatal encephalopathy following fetal distress. Arch Neurol 1976;33: 696–705.

Sarnat HB. Watershed infarcts in the fetal and neonatal brainstem. An aetiology of central hypoventilation, dysphagia, Moibius syndrome and micrognathia. Eur J Pediatr Neurol 2004;8:71–87.

Saugstad OD, Ramji S, Irani SF, et al. Resuscitation of newborn infants with 21% or 100% oxygen: Follow-up at 18 to 24 months. Pediatrics 2003;112:296–300.

Saugstad OD, Ramji S, Vento M. Resuscitation of depressed newborn infants with ambient air or pure oxygen: A meta-analysis. Biol Neonate 2004;87:27–34.

Shah P, Riphagen S, Beyenne J, et al. Multiorgan dysfunction in infants with post-asphyxial hypoxic-ischemic encephalopathy. Arch Dis Child Fetal Neonatal Ed 2004;89:F152–155.

Shankaran S. The postnatal management of the asphyxiated term infant. Clin Perinatol 2002;29:675.

Shankaran S, Laptook AR, Ehrenkranz RA, et al. Safety of whole body hypothermia for hypoxic-ischemic encephalopathy (HIE). Pediatr Res 2004;55:582A.

Sheth RD. Trends in the incidence and severity of intraventricular hemorrhage. Neurology 1998;13: 261–264.

Sie LT, van der Knaap MS, Oosting J, et al. MR patterns of hypoxic-ischemic brain damage after prenatal, perinatal or postnatal asphyxia. Neuropediatrics 2000;31:128–136.

Stevenson DK, Benitz WE, Sunshine P. Fetal and Neonatal Brain Injury: Mechanisms, Management and the Risks of Practice, 3rd edn. Cambridge: Cambridge University Press, 2003.

Taylor AG, Peter JC. Advantages of delayed VP shunting in posthemorrhagic hydrocephalus seen in low-birth-weight infants. Child's Nerv Syst 2001;17:328–333.

Vannucci RC, Towfighi J, Heitjan DF, et al. Carbon dioxide protects the perinatal brain from hypoxic-ischemic damage: An experimental study in the immature rat. Pediatrics 1995;95:868–874.

Vento M, Asensi M, Sastre J, et al. Hyperoxemia caused by resuscitation with pure oxygen may alter intracellular redox status by increasing oxidized glutathione in asphyxiated newly born infants. Semin Perinatol 2002;26:406–410.

Volpe JJ. Intracranial hemorrhage: germinal matrix – intraventricular hemorrhage of the premature infant. In: Neurology of the Newborn, 4th edn. Philadelphia: WB Saunders, 2000; p. 428.

Volpe JJ. Encephalopathy of prematurity includes neuronal abnormalities. Pediatrics 2005;116: 221–225.

Volpe JJ. Neurobiology of periventricular leukomalacia in the premature infant. Pediatr Res 2001;50: 553–562.

Whitelaw A. Repeated lumbar or ventricular punctures in newborns with intraventricular hemorrhage. Cochrane Database Syst Rev 2: CD000216; 2000.

Whitelaw A. Intraventricular streptokinase after intraventricular hemorrhage in newborn infants. Cochrane Database Syst Rev 1: CD 000498, 2001.

Whitelaw A, Kennedy CR and Brian LP. Diuretic therapy for newborn infants with posthemorrhagic ventricular dilatation. Cochrane Database Syst Rev 2: CD002270, 2001.

Wirrell EC, Armstrong EA, Osman LD and Yager JY. Prolonged seizures exacerbate perinatal hypoxic-ischemic brain damage. Pediatr Res 2001;50:445–454.

Yoon BH, Park CW and Chaiworapongsa T. Intrauterine infection and the development of cerebral palsy. BJOG 2003;110(Suppl. 20):124–127.

5

Trauma and Vascular Disorders

Gerald M. Fenichel

A birth-injured baby often generates feelings of guilt and bitter accusations of medical malpractice. Such injuries occur almost invariably against a background of either abnormal fetal presentation or difficult extraction, or both. The overall incidence of birth injuries is difficult to determine. Injuries vary not only from hospital to hospital, but even within the same hospital during different periods. In the United States, a decline in the incidence of cesarean section had changed the incidence of some birth injuries, especially brachial plexus injuries. Difficulties in labor and delivery of sufficient magnitude to cause birth injuries may also be associated with episodes of asphyxia. It is sometimes difficult to separate the relative importance of each factor's contribution to the resultant clinical state.

INJURIES TO THE SKULL AND SCALP

Cephalohematoma

- **Pathophysiology.** Cephalohematoma is an accumulation of blood confined to the subperiosteal space. It is always associated with underlying linear skull fractures.
- **Clinical features.** The hematoma forms a firm well-demarcated mass, almost invariably in a parietal location, that fails to extend across suture lines. Recognition of the mass occurs during the first 24 hours postpartum. Although cephalohematoma are more common on the right side than on the left, lateralization is unrelated to a right or left occiput position of the fetal head. Primiparity and forceps extraction are major risk factors. Depressed skull fractures are rare, but the false impression of depressed skull fracture is common, because palpation of the hematoma frequently reveals the presence of a recessed center in which there is a flat circular mass.

- **Diagnosis.** The basis for diagnosis is the clinical findings. Radiographic examination of the skull is unnecessary unless intracranial disease is suspected, then computed tomography (CT) is the best study to look for intracranial blood. Skull radiographs one month postpartum may suggest a depressed skull fracture because the periosteum, which is elevated over the hematoma, calcifies to form a circular opacity that resembles a bone edge.
- **Management.** Cephalohematomas require no treatment, resolve spontaneously within one month, and are not associated with chronic brain damage syndromes.

Subgaleal Hemorrhage

- **Pathophysiology.** A subgaleal hemorrhage is a collection of blood under the scalp. The subgaleal space, when distended 1 cm is capable of accepting 260 mL of blood. In the newborn, the volume of blood that can be lost in the subgaleal space is sufficient to produce anemia, shock, and death. The tearing of subcutaneous veins due to shearing forces applied during delivery causes the hemorrhage. Skull fractures, linear or depressed, are rarely associated. Important risk factors are vacuum extraction (Chenoy and Johnson, 1992), midforceps rotation, prolonged labor, and coagulopathies.
- **Clinical features.** The blood collects insidiously and may not be present until several hours or days after delivery. Blood tends to collect in a dependent position. The resulting mass is fluctuant.
- **Management.** The appearance of a subgaleal hemorrhage requires monitoring for the development of hypovolemic shock. All newborns with subgaleal hemorrhage require evaluation for coagulopathy and the administration of vitamin K. Transfusions of fresh whole blood are sometimes necessary. Spontaneous reabsorption of blood within a few weeks is the rule.

Skull Fracture

- **Pathophysiology.** Linear fractures of the skull usually heal completely within three months and are of no consequence to the child's future development. Depressed fractures of the skull are considerably less common than are linear fractures. Conditions that result in depressed fracture are extreme molding of the skull and the use of excessive force in the application of forceps. The depression can vary in size from a small dent 1 cm in diameter, which requires no therapy, to a major displacement of the frontal or parietal bone. As in cephalohematoma, the most common site of fracture is the right parietal bone. Depressed skull fractures in the newborn are similar to greenstick fractures of long bones because the continuity of the bone is uninterrupted.
- **Clinical features.** A rare complication of linear skull fracture is leptomeningeal cyst. Formation of a leptomeningeal cyst requires protrusion of the arachnoid through a defect produced by laceration of the dura and fracture of the skull. This most often occurs after vacuum extractions

(Djientcheu et al., 1996). The cyst presents as a pulsating mass within the scalp approximately three months after the time of fracture. Clear cerebrospinal fluid fills the cyst. With depressed skull fractures, the surface of the skull indents without cracking. The fracture does not extend beyond suture lines but will cause considerable separation of the adjacent sutures.

- **Management.** Linear fractures without leptomeningeal cysts require no treatment. Leptomeningeal cysts require surgical excision. If left in place, the cyst continues to grow and will cause a continuing separation of the fracture line. A second complication of untreated leptomeningeal cyst is irritation of the underlying cortex with generation of a focus for seizure activity. Most depressed fractures will elevate spontaneously over a period of months.

Intracranial Hemorrhage

Only a small percentage of fatal intracranial hemorrhage is attributable to trauma. Traumatic hemorrhages are mainly venous in origin and result from the tearing of either the dural sinuses or superficial veins or both. Blood accumulates in the subdural or subarachnoid spaces and may be supratentorial or infratentorial in location. Infratentorial subdural hematoma is a consequence of both laceration of the falx or tentorium and diastatic fracture of the occipital bone. By contrast, hemorrhages from asphyxia are virtually never subdural or intratentorial in location. Exceptions are intraventricular hemorrhage of the premature, which may cause hemorrhages into the cerebellum and petechial hemorrhages of the brainstem caused by herniation.

A hemorrhagic diathesis may occur in newborns of mothers treated with drugs that reduce vitamin K-dependent clotting factors or have genetic disturbances in the coagulation cascade. Severe bleeding may take place in the skin and internal organs but rarely into intracranial spaces. Administration of vitamin K reverses drug-induced bleeding and fresh frozen plasma corrects most genetic disturbances of clotting factors.

Intracranial hemorrhage and cerebral ischemia complicates the use of extracorporeal membrane oxygenation (ECHMO) in term newborns with pulmonary failure (Lago et al., 1995). Most are hemorrhagic or a combination of hemorrhagic and ischemic and some are purely ischemic.

Extradural Hemorrhage

- **Pathophysiology.** In children and adults, the typical cause of extradural hemorrhage is skull fracture by tearing of the middle meningeal artery in its groove within the temporal bone. Newborns and infants rarely develop extradural hemorrhage because the middle meningeal artery, not yet been encased within the bone, moves freely away from displacements of the skull. However, extradural hemorrhage may occur in the newborn, in the absence of skull fracture, when an external blow causes the outer layer of

the dura to detach from the inner table of the skull. This most often occurs following a difficult forceps extraction.
- **Clinical features.** Cephalohematoma is usually associated. Usually, evidence of cerebral is present at birth, but signs of increased intracranial pressure may delay for several hours. The fontanelle bulges, and brainstem function progressively declines, leading to death.
- **Diagnosis.** CT of the skull readily shows fractures and the location of intracranial hemorrhage. A unilateral or bilateral collection of extradural blood overlies the frontal and temporal lobes.
- **Management.** Surgical removal of the blood is lifesaving.

Supratentorial Subdural Hemorrhage

- **Pathophysiology.** Subdural hemorrhage in newborns is unusual. Once blood enters the subdural space, the force against the bridging veins is intensified and propagates a cycle of tearing, bleeding, and tearing. Subdural hemorrhage is therefore a self-perpetuating injury. Blood in the subdural space usually spreads evenly over the superior surface of the hemispheres and, if dispersed well and small in volume, may not cause any clinical signs in the newborn.
- **Clinical features.** Large supratentorial collections of blood in the subdural space produce a generalized increase in intracranial pressure. The fontanelles bulge and separation of the cranial sutures only partially relieves the pressure. State of consciousness progressively declines. Focal and multifocal clonic seizures occur on the second or third day postpartum and often accompanied by focal motor deficits. If unrelieved by subdural tap, increased intracranial pressure causes tentorial herniation. Evidence of herniation includes unilateral pupillary dilation and progressive brainstem dysfunction. Retinal hemorrhages are usually present.

  Focal collections of subdural blood may form, and these tend to localize over the frontal and parietal lobes. Large collections have an immediate pressure effect that lead to herniation and early death. More often, the hemorrhage is small in volume and remains asymptomatic during the immediate postpartum period. Clinical features of intracranial tension – vomiting, tense fontanelle, enlarging head circumference, altered states of consciousness, irritability, failure to thrive, and seizures – become progressively severe over a period of days, weeks, or months.
- **Diagnosis.** CT readily identifies the presence and location of subdural hemorrhages.
- **Management.** Most supratentorial hemorrhages can be removed by serial subdural puncture. Some require surgical evacuation.

Infratentorial Subdural Hemorrhage

- **Pathophysiology.** Excessive vertical molding of the head in vertex presentation, anteroposterior elongation of the head in face and brow presentations, and prolonged delivery of the aftercoming head in breech presentations are capable of producing intolerable stress on the tentorium and falx. Forces of stress can produce a tear in the tentorium near its junction with the falx. The laceration is located at the site where the inferior sagittal sinus joins the great cerebral vein to form the straight sinus. Lacerations at this site, whether complete or incomplete, tear the tentorial arteries and large venous sinuses, causing hemorrhage into the subdural space of the posterior fossa and compression of the cerebellum downward against the medulla. Traumatic subarachnoid and intraparenchymal hemorrhages are often associated, as is an asphyxial encephalopathy. The lateral and medial foramina of the fourth ventricle, by which cerebrospinal fluid exits into the subarachnoid space, obliterates. If brainstem compression from the acute hemorrhage is not sufficient to cause death, hydrocephalus is the expected outcome in survivors.

- **Clinical features.** Small accumulations of infratentorial blood are often asymptomatic and seen using CT in many newborns following vacuum extractions. Large accumulations of blood cause clinical evidence of brainstem compression. Onset of symptoms may delay for 12 hours or longer following delivery. Alterations in the rate, depth, or rhythm of respirations occur first. Cry becomes abnormal, described as high-pitched or hoarse. Difficulty with feeding follows, due to vomiting and loss of the sucking reflex. Neurological decline is progressive and characterized by decreasing states of consciousness, hypotonia, and seizures. Pupillary dilation from third nerve palsy is unusual, but sixth nerve palsy, skew deviation of the eyes, and nystagmus are relatively common. Fontanelles are tense, and head circumference enlarges rapidly. Anemia can be associated.
- **Diagnosis.** Examination of the cerebrospinal fluid usually reveals bloody or xanthochromic fluid with marked elevation of the protein concentration. However, when suspecting intracranial hemorrhage, lumbar puncture is contraindicated and CT is the appropriate procedure for diagnosis. CT is superior to ultrasound for the demonstration of posterior fossa hemorrhage, supratentorial subarachnoid hemorrhage, and fractures of the occipital bone. *Occipital osteodiastasis*, a separation of the squamous and lateral portions of the occipital bone, may be associated with tentorial tear in term newborns delivered in breech position.
- **Management.** Large infratentorial subdural hemorrhages are always associated with prolonged difficult deliveries. Severe hypoxic-ischemic encephalopathy is usually associated. Removal of blood intracranial blood may not influence outcome.

Supratentorial Subarachnoid Hemorrhage

- **Pathophysiology.** It is easier to explain why some bleeding might occur over the cerebral convexities in every newborn born by vaginal delivery than why it might not. The skull of the newborn is pliable and easily displaced from the soft underlying brain. Numerous thin-walled veins, which drain the cortex by traversing the arachnoid to reach the venous sinuses enclosed in the dura, must undergo considerable deformity as the head molds in the birth canal. Normal molding forces on the skull are of sufficient magnitude to rupture these delicate bridging vessels and cause hemorrhage into the subarachnoid and subdural spaces.

- **Clinical features.** Subarachnoid hemorrhage may be focal or diffuse. Focal subarachnoid hemorrhage usually overlies a cerebral infarction and the discussion is later in this chapter. Diffuse subarachnoid hemorrhage occurs in term newborns following a long labor and difficult delivery. Such newborns usually have some degree of intrauterine asphyxia but do not have severe hypoxic-ischemic encephalopathy. After initial resuscitation, they appear well until seizures occur.
- **Diagnosis.** CT shows blood in the interhemispheric fissure and in supratentorial and infratentorial recesses. Many of these newborns will have a normal outcome.
- **Management.** Management is supportive.

Intracerebral Hemorrhage

- **Pathophysiology.** Primary intracerebral hemorrhages in term newborns are unilateral and usually parietal or temporal in location. Trauma and hemorrhagic infarction account for isolated intraparenchymal hemorrhage in some newborns, and hyperviscosity, arteriovenous malformation, coagulopathy, and tumor are identifiable causes in rare cases. In many, the mechanism underlying the hemorrhage is not identifiable. Temporal lobe hemorrhage, like parietal lobe hemorrhage, may be of uncertain etiology, and occurs after applying excessive force to the temporal portion of the skull by obstetrical forceps. The latter is now uncommon. When forceps are causative, contusion of the scalp overlying the area and linear fracture of the skull is present.
- **Clinical features.** Parietal and frontoparietal hemorrhages are often of uncertain cause. Such newborns are usually normal at birth and appear well until the onset of seizures, usually focal, during the first week. Focal clonic seizures always indicate a cerebral infarction or hemorrhage. With time, focal encephalomalacia replaces the area of hemorrhage. Contralateral hemiplegia is an expected outcome but the severity of the weakness may be difficult to predict. Temporal lobe hemorrhage is associated with altered states of consciousness, hemiparesis contralateral to the hematoma, and focal or generalized seizures.
- **Diagnosis.** Newborns with focal clonic seizures should be evaluated immediately using CT or ultrasound to look for intracerebral hemorrhage. If the CT is normal, magnetic resonance imaging (MRI) done 3 days later reveals cerebral infarction.
- **Management.** Anticonvulsant therapy and general supportive measures are required. The infarcted space may eventually result in a porencephalic cyst.

Intracerebellar Hemorrhage

- **Pathophysiology.** Term newborns with intracerebellar hemorrhage are usually the product of a difficult labor and delivery. In prematures,

intracerebellar hemorrhage is associated with periventricular-intraventricular hemorrhage (see Ch. 4).
- **Clinical features.** Apneic spells and hypotonia occur soon after birth. The fontanelle is tense and the cerebrospinal fluid is bloody. Mental retardation, hypotonia, and cerebellar ataxia are the expected features in survivors.
- **Diagnosis.** CT or ultrasound shows the hemorrhage.
- **Management.** Surgical evacuation of the hematoma relieves pressure in the posterior fossa.

Intraventricular Hemorrhage at Term

- **Pathophysiology.** Intraventricular hemorrhage in prematures is relatively common and is associated with the respiratory distress syndrome (see Ch. 4). Intraventricular hemorrhage in term newborns is uncommon and multifactorial. Some bleeds occur weeks after birth. The hemorrhage may originate in the subependymal matrix, the choroid plexus, or both.
- **Clinical features.** More than half of intraventricular hemorrhages occur in newborns delivered with difficulty, frequently from breech position, and have suffered some degree of intrauterine asphyxia. The babies show bruises and evidence of distress at birth. Resuscitation is required and despite the appearance of improvement, multifocal seizures occur at 24 to 48 hours. The cerebrospinal fluid is bloody and the fontanelle may be tense. Many of these children will have permanent neurological handicaps. Intraventricular hemorrhage also occurs in term newborns with no history of either trauma or asphyxia. Such newborns appear normal at birth, have excellent Apgar scores, and develop spells of apnea and cyanosis in the first hours or days after birth.
- **Diagnosis.** CT or ultrasound shows the hemorrhage (Heibel et al., 1993). Selected newborns with either a family history of bleeding disorders or no history of a difficult delivery require coagulation studies.
- **Management.** Most require the same management techniques described for intraventricular hemorrhage in the premature. Posthemorrhagic hydrocephalus is common. Among all term newborns with intraventricular hemorrhage, 35% will require shunt placement.

SPINAL CORD INJURIES

Spinal cord injuries are uncommon. They cord occur when nonphysiological forces are applied to the head and neck of the fetus. Approximately 75% of such injuries are associated with vaginal delivery of a breech presentation; the other 25% are associated with vaginal delivery of a cephalic presentation. Spinal cord injuries are almost unheard of in fetuses delivered by cesarean section. In breech presentation, the damage is most often located in the lower cervical and upper thoracic regions and results from excessive stretching of the cord by traction. With cephalic presentation, the site of damage is the higher cervical segments, and the usual mechanism of injury is by twisting of the neck during mid-forceps rotation. Injuries of the lower thoracic and lumbar spinal cord are even less common and usually related to vascular occlusion secondary to umbilical artery catheterization or air embolus from peripheral intravenous injection.

Hemorrhage into the posterior fossa and avulsion of the brachial plexus may accompany severe traction or rotational injuries. These are not compatible with survival. By contrast, mild traction injuries could cause edema of the spinal cord without disrupting its anatomical continuity and without jeopardizing survival. Such injuries might produce little or no clinical disturbance in the newborn. The only symptom is mild, generalized hypotonia, often falsely attributed to asphyxia resulting from a difficult labor and delivery.

Spinal Cord Injuries in Breech Presentation

- **Pathophysiology.** Spinal cord injury among newborns delivered in breech position occurs almost exclusively when the angle of extension of the fetal head exceeds 90 degrees; the risk of spinal cord injury in this group is greater than 70%. The causes of intrauterine hyperextension of the head and neck are sometimes an underlying congenital malformation of the cervical vertebrae or generalized hypotonia, but most often, the cause of hyperextension is uncertain. Whether or not an underlying defect is present, the hyperextended posture markedly increases the vulnerability of the cervical spine to traction injuries. The time of greatest danger is during delivery. The longitudinal forces applied to the extended head are sufficient not only to stretch the cord but also herniates the brainstem through the foramen magnum. Every fetus in breech presentation with a 90-degree angle of head extension requires delivery by cesarean section.

  Postmortem examination of newborns with spinal cord traction injuries demonstrates epidural, subdural, and intramedullary hemorrhages, which are most extensive in the lower cervical and upper thoracic segments, but may extend the entire length of the spinal cord. Hemorrhage and laceration of the paravertebral muscles occur as well. Concurrent hemorrhage into the posterior fossa and laceration of the cerebellum is secondary to occipital osteodiastasis, tentorial tear, and traction herniation of the cerebellum and brainstem through the foramen magnum.
- **Clinical features.** Newborns with brainstem injuries are unconscious and atonic at birth; survival beyond the immediate neonatal period is rare. Injuries restricted to the low cervical and high thoracic segments of the spinal cord present as flaccid quadriplegia or diplegia with diaphragmatic breathing. Movement in the proximal muscles of the arms is relatively normal, and there may be flexion at the elbows if the biceps are of near-normal strength (C5) and are unopposed by weak triceps (C6). A pistol posture of the hand occurs in which the thumb and forefinger extend and the other three digits flex. Spontaneous movement of the legs is absent, but a withdrawal reflex to pinprick (a spinal cord reflex generated by an isolated lower segment) is present after spinal shock has subsided. The bladder distends and urine dribbles. A sensory level to pinprick is established when the child's state of

alertness permits detailed testing. In the obtunded newborn, the absence of sweating below the level of injury indicates the level.

- **Diagnosis.** MRI of the spinal cord shows the extent of the injury.
- **Management.** Management is the same as for spinal cord injuries at any age.

Spinal Cord Injuries in Cephalic Presentation

- **Pathophysiology.** Spinal cord injuries associated with cephalic presentation result from torsion rather than from traction of the spinal cord. Such injuries usually occur during a midforceps rotation in which the trunk fails to rotate with the head. The absence of amniotic fluid, secondary to delay in applying forceps after rupture of the membranes, increases the risk of failure for rotation of the trunk with the head. Because midforceps are most likely to be applied after prolonged labor that has progressed poorly, cerebral disturbances from trauma, asphyxia, or both may be expected as well. The most severe injury is transection of the cord at the level of the odontoid process caused by fracture of the odontoid. Postmortem examination demonstrates discontinuity of the cord with epidural and subarachnoid hemorrhages at the C1 and C2 levels.
- **Clinical features.** Newborns with cord transection are flaccid and fail to breathe spontaneously. Eye movements and the suck reflex are present, but movement of the limbs, except for the withdrawal reflex, is lacking. Sweating is absent over the entire body, and priapism may be present. The high cervical injury obviates any change for the establishment of spontaneous respiration. Death quickly follows discontinuation of mechanical ventilation. With milder injuries, the intracranial structures are undisturbed, and there is no evidence of epidural hemorrhage in the cord. Instead, multiple petechial hemorrhages, which may localize to the posterior horns or columns, are present in the high cervical region. Although newborns are apneic at birth, some develop spontaneous but labored respiration later. The cranial nerves function normally, but flaccid paralysis and analgesia are complete in all limbs. Death from respiratory complications usually follows within the first week, although some children have survived for many years with varying degrees of handicaps.
- **Diagnosis.** MRI of the spinal cord shows the extent of the injury.
- **Management.** Management is the same as for spinal cord injuries at any age.

Postnatal Spinal Cord Injury

Acute and sometimes irreversible paraplegia may occur in newborns after umbilical artery catheterization. The cause of the paraplegia is infarction of the spinal cord secondary to embolism in the artery of Adamkiewicz. This artery arises from the aorta, at the T10 to T12 level of the aorta and is the major segmental artery to the thoracolumbar cord. In cases of cord infarction, the placement of the umbilical catheter tip was between T8 and T11. Lower placement avoids the complication, but causes a higher incidence of ischemia to the legs.

Transverse myelopathy from compressive hematoma is a rare event after the onset of sepsis with disseminated intravascular coagulation. Spontaneous movement in all limbs is lost as are tendon reflexes in all limbs. Neurological features include depressed pinprick sensation below the neck, paradoxical respirations, and a neurogenic bladder.

FACIAL NERVE ASYMMETRIES

Most facial asymmetries observed at birth result from congenital aplasia of muscle and not from trauma. Muscle aplasia is the usual cause of facial diplegia. Complete unilateral palsies are likely to be traumatic in origin, while partial unilateral palsies may be either traumatic or aplastic.

Traumatic Facial Nerve Palsy

- **Pathophysiology.** Traumatic facial nerve palsy is very uncommon. The highest incidence is in term newborns delivered at term in cephalic presentation. A relationship exists between the side of the facial palsy and the obstetrical position. Fetuses that lie in occipitoleft positions have left facial palsies; fetuses that lie in occipitoright positions have right facial palsies. The implication of this relationship between occipital position and side of facial palsy is that traumatic facial nerve palsies in the newborn are the result of nerve compression against the sacrum during labor and not of the misapplications of forceps. While the use of mid-forceps in difficult deliveries may cause permanent facial palsy, even in this group, intrauterine factors are equally important (Hamish et al., 1996; Shapiro et al., 1996).
- **Clinical features.** The clinical expression of complete unilateral facial palsy in the newborn can be subtle and need not be apparent immediately after birth. Failure of eye closure on the affected side is the first sign that calls attention to the weakness. Only when the child cries does a flaccid paralysis of all facial muscles become obvious. The eyeball rolls up behind the open lid, the nasolabial fold remains flat, and the corner of the mouth does not pull down. Indeed, because only the normal side of the mouth droops during crying, the normal side may be thought to be paralyzed and the paralyzed side normal.

  When there is partial paralysis of the facial nerve, the orbicularis oculi is the muscle most frequently spared. In these injuries, the site of compression is usually over the parotid gland with sparing of nerve fibers that course upward just after leaving the stylomastoid foramen. Unilateral, isolated weakness of the depressor anguli oris muscle (DAOM) should be considered a separate and specific entity caused by congenital aplasia of muscle rather than trauma.
- **Diagnosis.** The diagnosis is based on the clinical examination.
- **Management.** No prospective studies are available that report the natural outcome of facial nerve injuries that occurred at birth. Most investigators

are optimistic and indicate a high rate of spontaneous recovery. The optimism may be warranted, but it is based on anecdotal experience alone. In the absence of data on long-term outcome, it is impossible to evaluate the efficacy of any therapeutic measures that have been suggested. In most newborns, it is reasonable to caution against surgical intervention except when the nerve is lacerated. In that event, it makes sense to reconstitute the nerve, if possible, or at least to allow the proximal stump a clear pathway toward regeneration by debridement of the wound.

Congenital Hypoplasia of Facial Muscles

Aplasia of Facial Muscles

- **Pathophysiology.** The site of pathology in the Möbius syndrome is usually the facial nerve nuclei and their internuclear connections (Jaradeh et al., 1996). The abnormal gene in one family with dominantly inherited Möbius syndrome was mapped to the long arm of chromosome 3. Other developmental causes of unilateral facial palsy are Goldenhar's syndrome, the Poland anomoly, DiGeorge syndrome, osteopetrosis, and trisomy 13 and 18 (Shapiro et al., 1996).
- **Clinical features.** Facial diplegia may occur alone, with bilateral abducens palsies, or with involvement of several cranial nerves. Congenital malformations elsewhere in the body—dextrocardia, talipes equinovarus, absent pectoral muscle, and limb deformities—may be associated.
- **Diagnosis.** MRI of the brain is indicated in all such cases of congenital facial diplegia to determine whether other cerebral malformations are present. Causes other than primary malformation must be considered as well. Electromyography (EMG) can help determine the timing of injury. Denervation potentials are present only if the facial nuclei or nerves were injured 2 to 6 weeks before the study. Facial muscles that are aplastic as a result of Möbius syndrome or nerve injury occurring early in gestation do not show active denervation.
- **Management.** Surgical procedures are being developed that provide partial facial movement.

Depressor Anguli Oris Muscle Aplasia

- **Clinical features.** Isolated unilateral weakness of the depressor anguli oris muscle (DAOM) is the most common cause of facial asymmetry at birth. One corner of the mouth fails to move downward when the child cries. All other facial movements are symmetrical. The lower lip on the paralyzed side feels thinner to palpation, even at birth, suggesting antepartum hypoplasia.
- **Diagnosis.** Traumatic lesions of the facial nerve would not selectively injure nerve fibers to the DAOM and spare all other facial muscles. Electrodiagnostic studies help differentiate aplasia of the DAOM from

traumatic facial injury. In aplasia the conduction velocity and latency of the facial nerve are normal. Fibrillations are not present at the site of the DAOM. Instead, motor unit potentials are absent or decreased in number.
- **Management.** No treatment is available or needed. The DAOM is not a significant component of facial expression in older children and adults, and its absence is hardly noticed.

Brachial Plexus Palsy

Traumatic Brachial Plexus Palsy

- **Pathophysiology.** Obstetrical brachial plexus palsies are caused by excessive traction. The upper plexus is injured when the head is suddenly pulled away from the arm. This occurs, in vertex position when the head is forcefully pulled to deliver the aftercoming shoulder or when the head and neck are forced downward by normal contractions while the shoulder is caught in the pelvis. Injuries in breech position occur when the arm is pulled downward to free the after-coming head or when the head is rotated to occipitoanterior, but the shoulder is fixed. Complete (upper and lower) plexus injuries occur during vertex deliveries when traction is exerted on a prolapsed arm and in breech deliveries when the trunk is pulled downward but an aftercoming arm is fixed. The important elements that increase the risk of injury are a primiparous mother, a term newborn of normal or heavy weight, a prolonged and difficult delivery, and malposition of the fetus.

  Brachial plexus injuries are reported as occurring in utero secondary to malposition of the fetus (Gherman et al., 1999). Such occurrences are exceedingly uncommon and the possibility of a hereditary brachial plexus palsy should always be considered (see next section).
- **Clinical features.** It is traditional to divide brachial plexus palsies into those involving the upper roots (C5, C6) and those involving the lower roots (C8, T1); the former palsies are named after *Erb* and *Duchenne* and the latter after *Klumpke*. In fact, solitary lower root injuries rarely occur at birth. The fifth and sixth cervical roots are constantly affected; the seventh cervical root is also involved in 50% of injuries; and total brachial plexus paralysis, involving all roots from C5 to T1, occurs in 10% of injuries. Bilateral, but not necessarily symmetrical, involvement occurs in 8% to 23% of cases. Damage to the lower roots is sometimes associated with Horner's syndrome, while injuries that extend higher than the fourth cervical segment may result in ipsilateral diaphragmatic and hypoglossal paralysis. Because the upper plexus (C5 to C7) is almost always involved, the posture of the arm is typical and reflects weakness of the proximal muscles. The arm is abducted and internally rotated at the shoulder and is extended and pronated at the elbow, so that the partially flexed fingers face backward. Extension of the wrist is lost and the fingers are fisted. The biceps and triceps reflexes are absent. Injuries that extend higher than the C4 segment result in ipsilateral diaphragmatic paralysis. Newborns with complete brachial plexus palsies have flaccid, dry limbs with neither proximal nor distal movement.

A Horner syndrome is sometimes associated. Sensory loss to pinprick is present with partial or complete palsies but may not conform to the segmental pattern of weakness. Associated with brachial plexus injuries are an increased incidence of asphyxia, facial nerve palsy, and fractures of the clavicle and humerus.

- **Diagnosis.** Brachial plexus palsy is easily recognized by the typical posture of the arm and by failure of movement when the Moro reflex is tested. Because the injury often takes place during a long and difficult delivery, asphyxia may be present as well. In such cases focal arm weakness may be missed because of generalized hypotonia. Approximately 10% of newborns with brachial plexus injuries have facial nerve palsy and fractures of the clavicle or humerus.
- **Management.** Spontaneous recovery rates are approximately 70–90%. Those that show improvement in the first month have the best prognosis. One goal of therapy is to prevent the development of contractures. Range-of-motion exercises should be started in the first week after birth and continued thereafter. Splinting should be avoided. Contractures develop quickly and may cause permanent disability even when the nerves are recovered. Surgical reconstruction of the plexus (nerve grafts, neuroma excision, etc.) is a consideration in infants with no evidence of spontaneous recovery at 6 months (Laurent and Lee, 1994). However, the benefit of reconstructive surgery is not established.

Genetic Brachial Plexus Palsy

- **Pathophysiology.** Genetic abnormalities of myelin should be considered in newborns with brachial plexus palsy following cesarean section, easy vaginal deliveries, or those with a family history of brachial plexus palsy. The disorder is transmitted by autosomal dominant inheritance and the gene maps to 17q25 (Stögbauer et al., 2000).
- **Clinical features.** Hereditary brachial plexopathy is difficult to distinguish from traumatic brachial plexus palsy in the absence of a family history.
- **Diagnosis.** DNA-based diagnosis is available.
- **Management.** Ranges of motion exercises are recommended.

OTHER NERVE INJURIES

Isolated peripheral nerve injuries in the newborn are most often caused by pressure, often iatrogenic, sometimes during labor.

Radial Nerve Injuries

- **Pathophysiology.** Most cases involve a prolonged or difficult labor in which there was pressure of the radial nerve proximal to the radial epicondyle of the humerus. Some of the injuries may actually occur before the onset of labor. Postpartum radial nerve injury may occur in prematures following repeated ultrasound measurements of blood pressure in the same area.

- **Clinical features.** Radial nerve injuries cause flaccid paralysis of the wrist and finger extensors. Localized pressure necrosis of the subcutaneous fat is often present as well.
- **Diagnosis.** The clinical features establish the diagnosis. EMG may be useful to date the timing of injury.
- **Management.** Spontaneous recovery is the rule in newborns with isolated pressure palsies of the radial nerve. Range of motion exercises are recommended.

Medial Nerve Injuries

- **Pathophysiology.** Medial nerve injuries are uncommon but may result when arterial gas samples are obtained at the anticubital fossa and at the wrist.
- **Clinical features.** Proximal injuries produce decreased flexion of all fingers, while distal injuries mainly affect the thumb. Both may result in permanent impairment of pincer movements.
- **Diagnosis.** The clinical features establish the diagnosis. EMG may be useful to date the timing of injury.
- **Management.** Range of motion exercises are recommended.

Isolated Peroneal Nerve Injuries

- **Pathophysiology.** Isolated peroneal nerve injury may occur intrapartum from pressure on the nerve (Jones et al., 1996) and postpartum from pressure from the use of footboards or the infiltration of intravenous fluids.
- **Clinical features.** The presenting feature is foot drop. Those that occur intrapartum tend to resolve spontaneously.
- **Diagnosis.** The clinical features establish the diagnosis. EMG may be useful to date the timing of injury.
- **Management.** A splint that holds the foot in neutral position will avoid contracture of the heel cord while the nerves are recovering.

CEREBRAL INFARCTION

- **Pathophysiology.** Cerebral infarction from arterial occlusion occurs more often at term than in prematures. Underlying conditions that predispose to infarction include sepsis related disseminated intravascular coagulation (DIC), polycythemia, respiratory distress, cardiac surgery, and maternal cocaine use. The combination of DIC and sepsis is associated with multiple small infarcts, while respiratory distress syndrome and cardiac surgery are usually associated with single large infarcts but also may cause multiple infarcts. A single large infarction can occur during the course of a difficult delivery when there is physical injury to the carotid or middle cerebral arteries.

- **Clinical features.** The clinical picture of arterial infarction secondary to DIC is hypotonia, lethargy, cardiovascular collapse, and death. Focal neurological signs are not present, and seizures are uncommon. Most will die within the first week if the disorder is not promptly reversed. Newborns with single, unilateral infarcts appear normal at birth and generally have no risk factors for infarction. Seizures, usually focal motor, develop during the first 2 weeks postpartum. Neurological examination may be normal initially. Neurological outcome is generally good when the infarct is small. Larger infarcts, especially those that become porencephalic, are associated with some degree of hemiparesis. Seizures may persist into childhood, even when motor function is normal.
- **Diagnosis.** Large infarcts in the distribution of the middle cerebral artery can be detected by ultrasound. CT or MRI is needed to detect small unilateral infarcts. The infarction is usually frontal or parietal in location and more often in the left hemisphere than in the right. Subarachnoid hemorrhage may overlie the area of infarction.
- **Management.** Newborns with unilateral infarcts and seizures are treated with phenobarbital for the first month. After a month, it is reasonable to stop treatment if electroencephalography does not show epileptiform activity. Those with evidence of hemiparesis should be referred for physical therapy.

Vascular Anomalies

Intracranial arteriovenous malformations and arterial aneurysms are uncommon in the newborn. They are discussed in this chapter because they are sometimes considered in the differential diagnosis of intracranial hemorrhage. Subarachnoid hemorrhage in the newborn from aneurysmal rupture is a rare occurrence, but hemorrhage from arteriovenous malformations is exceptional during the first month postpartum. A more important consideration in the differential diagnosis of intracranial hemorrhage in the newborn is a bleeding disposition caused by defective coagulation. Such defects may be secondary to systemic disorders (i.e. thrombocytopenia and DIC related to sepsis and/or asphyxia) or vitamin K deficiency (i.e. newborns whose mothers were treated with anticoagulants or phenytoin during pregnancy). Primary genetic disturbances in the mechanism of coagulation rarely present during the immediate newborn period as intracranial hemorrhage.

Arteriovenous Malformations

- **Pathophysiology.** The cerebral vasculature originates from a germinal bed of blood-containing channels that cannot be identified as either arteries or veins. This germinal bed, located at the base of the brain, forms a network that covers the developing brain before differentiating further into arteries, capillaries, and veins. A cerebral circulation is established by 5 weeks' gestation, the arteries are identifiable at 2 months and the veins at 3 months. As arteriovenous malformations are abnormalities of this process, they must originate early in embryonic life. Several different arteriovenous malformations of the cerebral circulation may become symptomatic during infancy and childhood, but only malformations of the *great vein of Galen* becomes symptomatic in the newborn.

The malformation may be a simple varix, but most are complex anastomoses that have been likened to a bag of worms. Feeding vessels are countless in number and vary in structure from well-differentiated arteries to malformed unclassifiable vessels. The surrounding brain parenchyma becomes necrotic from ischemia as blood is stolen by the malformation, from hemorrhagic infarction caused by thrombosis within the malformation, and from compression by the growing mass (Lasjaunias et al., 1996; Meyers et al., 2000).

- **Clinical features.** Eighty percent of newborns with malformations of the great vein of Galen are males. Most often, medical attention is sought not for symptoms of intracranial pathology, but rather because of high-output cardiac failure. The typical initial diagnosis is cyanotic congenital heart disease. Radiographs of the chest show an enlarged heart that is normal in shape. The cardiac enlargement may prompt catheterization. It is often during this procedure that the diagnosis of cerebral arteriovenous malformation is established. The aortic vessels destined for the brain are enlarged in size, and the superior vena cava opacifies rapidly and contains blood that has a higher than normal oxygen saturation. A cranial bruit is invariably present; unexplained persistent hypoglycemia is sometimes noted.

In addition to the cardiac symptomology, some newborns may also demonstrate rapid enlargement of the head, although this symptom is more commonly encountered in infancy. Megalencephaly may occur, in part, as a result of the increased intracranial volume of the mass, but the more important factor is hydrocephalus. The arteriovenous malformation, by its position just above the quadrigeminal plate, compresses the aqueduct and causes dilation of the lateral ventricles. Hemorrhage is almost unheard of in the newborn and rarely occurs during infancy.

A direct surgical approach to the malformation is rarely possible. Not only is the mortality rate high, but the hope for adequate brain function in survivors is already limited by the pre-existing damage to the brain by the malformation. Embolization of the malformation is now considered the treatment of choice. The long-term results of embolization are not yet known.

Arterial Aneurysm

Aneurysms are vestiges of the embryonic circulation and tend to be located, in postnatal life, at the bifurcation of major arteries. Ruptured intracranial aneurysms are exceptionally rare throughout childhood: only five instances have been documented in the newborn (Grode et al., 1978; Lee et al., 1978). In two, the rupture occurred immediately after birth, and in the other three, it was delayed until the third and fourth weeks. In two of the five children, the diagnosis was made at postmortem examination. Failure of antemortem diagnosis rests simply with the failure to consider the possibility of arterial aneurysm; the technology for diagnosis is certainly available by arteriography.

The symptoms are those of subarachnoid hemorrhage. The presentation may be catastrophic (sudden loss of consciousness, tachycardia, hypotension, a bulging fontanelle, and generalized depression of tone) but more often is subtle. The initial symptoms are episodes of apnea and decreased feeding. Alterations in consciousness and increasing fullness of the fontanelle follow. The finding of grossly bloody or xanthochromic *cerebrospinal fluid* on lumbar puncture confirms the occurrence of a subarachnoid hemorrhage. Precise diagnosis and localization of the aneurysm are sometimes possible with contrast-enhanced CT, but usually requires arteriography. In two patients, the aneurysm was attached to the middle cerebral artery and could be successfully clipped. No objective evidence of residual neurological disturbance was present postoperatively in either child. In the other three patients, the aneurysms originated in the basilar system near the junction of the inferior cerebellar artery, and the hemorrhages proved fatal.

REFERENCES

Chenoy R and Johnson R. A randomized prospective study comparing delivery with metal and silicone rubber vacuum extractor cups. Br J Obstet Gynaecol 1992;99:360–363.

Djientcheu VD, Rilliet B, Delavelle J, et al. Leptomeningeal cyst in newborns due to vacuum extraction: report of two cases. Child Nerv Syst 1996;12:399–403.

Gherman RB, Ouzounian JG and Goodwin TM. Brachial plexus palsy: an in utero injury. Am J Obstet Gynecol 1999;180:1303–1307.

Grode ML, Saunders M and Carton CA. Subarachnoid hemorrhage secondary to ruptured aneurysms in infants. J Neurosurg 1978;49:898–902.

Hamish J, Laing E, Harrison DH, et al. Arch Dis Child 1996;74:56–58.

Heibel M, Heber R, Bechinger D, et al. Early diagnosis of perinatal cerebral lesions in apparently normal full-term newborns by ultrasound of the brain. Neuroradiology 1993;35:85–91.

Jaradeh S, D'Cruz O, Howard JF Jr, et al. Mobius syndrome: Electrophysiologic studies in seven cases. Muscle Nerve 1996;19:1148–1153.

Jones HR, Herbison GJ, Jacobs SR, et al. Muscle Nerve 1996;19:88–91.

Lago P, Rebsamen S, Clancy RR, et al. MRI, MRA and neurodevelopmental outcome following neonatal ECMO. Pediatr Neurol 1995;12:294–305.

Lasjaunias PL, Alvarez H, Rodesch G, et al. Aneurysmal malformations of the vein of Galen. Intervent Neuroradiol 1996;2:15–26.

Laurent JP and Lee R. Birth-related upper brachial plexus injuries in infants: operative and nonoperative approaches. J Child Neurol 1994;9:111–117.

Lee YL, Kandall SR and Ghali VS. Intracerebral arterial aneurysm in a newborn. Arch Neurol 1978;74:268–270.

Meyers PM, Halbach VV, Phatouros CP, et al. Hemorrhagic complications in vein of Galen malformations. Ann Neurol 2000;47:748–755.

Shapiro NL, Cunningham MJ, Parikh SJ, et al. Congenital unilateral facial palsy. Pediatrics 1996;98: 261–265.

Stögbauer F, Young P, Kuhlenbaumer G, et al. Hereditary recurrent focal neuropathies. Clinical and molecular features. Neurology 2000;54:546–551.

6

Infectious Diseases

Jörn-Hendrik Weitkamp
and Joseph J. Nania

This chapter is limited in scope to the more common intrauterine and perinatal infections that affect the nervous system. Infections may occur by transplacental infection, during labor and delivery, and in the nursery, especially among extremely premature newborns requiring indwelling catheters and invasive procedures. Maternal infection, the source of transplacental fetal infection, is often undiagnosed during pregnancy. Neurological diseases caused by these infections may include meningitis, encephalitis, myelitis, or malformations of the central nervous system.

VIRUSES

CYTOMEGALOVIRUS

Congenital cytomegalovirus (CMV) infection is a major cause of neurological sequelae and one of the most common causes of hearing loss in the United States. CMV is an enveloped double-stranded DNA virus and the largest member of the herpesvirus group. CMV tends to produce chronic infections with typical cytopathology of enlarged (cytomegalic) cells containing cytoplasmic and intranuclear inclusions.

Epidemiology

CMV is highly species specific and transmitted from person to person through virus-containing secretions, from mother to infant before, during, or after birth, and by blood products from previously infected people (Stagno, 2001). CMV persists in latent form after a primary infection, and reactivation can occur years later, particularly under conditions of immunosuppression.

CMV infection, the most common congenital infection in humans, causes severe injury to the infected fetus. Risks to the fetus are greatest during the first half of gestation. The rate of CMV acquisition in childbearing-aged women is approximately 2–6% per year with higher rates among women of lower socioeconomic background. Most serum-negative women acquire CMV from exposure to toddlers, who attend group day care. Up to 70% of children between 1 and 3 years attending group day care, shed CMV. Congenital CMV infection occurs in 0.2 and 2% of all newborns in the United States because of both primary and recurrent maternal infection. Intrauterine transmission can take place in 30 to 40% of births after primary maternal infection in contrast to only 0.9 to 1.5% after recurrent infection. The risk for symptomatic disease and sequelae is also highest after primary maternal infection and in premature infants.

Perinatal infection occurs through maternal shedding of CMV in the genital tract and/or breast milk. Cervical shedding near term takes place in about 10% of women and intrapartum transmission rates are 2.5%. CMV excretion into breast milk occurs in approximately 14% of immediate postpartum women and transmission of CMV via breast milk occurs in 5 to 15% of cases.

Postnatal infection of otherwise healthy infants with CMV rarely results in symptomatic disease. However, symptomatic disease and even death follow transmission of CMV via blood products in serum-negative premature neonates. Transmission of CMV through breast-feeding in extremely premature infants may cause hepatic dysfunction and sepsis-like symptoms. However, postnatal ingestion of CMV-positive milk by either premature or term infants is not associated with long-term developmental or hearing impairments.

Infants with congenital or perinatally acquired CMV shed virus consistently into saliva for 2–4 years and into urine for up to 6 years. The highest quantities of virus excretion are in the first six months of life, and symptomatically infected children shed virus in larger quantities than do asymptomatic infants.

Clinical Features

Approximately 10% of the estimated 44,000 CMV-infected infants born in the United States each year are symptomatic at birth. Clinical manifestations include intrauterine growth retardation, jaundice, petechiae/purpura, hepatosplenomegaly, microcephaly, hydrocephaly, intracerebral calcifications, glaucoma, and chorioretinitis. Table 6–1 lists these clinical manifestations and their frequency of occurrence compared to other congenital infections, such as rubella, toxoplasmosis, and syphilis. Pneumonitis, a common clinical manifestation of CMV infection after renal or bone marrow transplant in adults, occurs rarely in congenitally infected infants. Except for the brain, most organ involvement is self-limited.

The most frequently noted presenting signs of congenital CMV disease are a generalized petechial rash, hepatosplenomegaly, and jaundice.

- **Petechiae/purpura.** Depression of platelet formation is a direct effect of CMV on megakaryocytes in the bone marrow. Petechiae are not usually

TABLE 6–1   Clinical manifestations of common congenital infections*

Sign	CMV	Rubella	Toxoplasmosis	Syphilis
Hepatoslenomegaly	++	+	+	+
Jaundice	+	+	+	+
Exanthem	−	−	+	++
Petechiae/purpura	++	+	+	+
Hydrocephalus	+	−	++	−
Microcephalus	++	−	+	−
Intracerebral calcifications	++	−	++	−
Heart defects	−	++	−	−
Bone lesions	−	++	−	++
Glaucoma	−	+	−	+
Intrauterine growth retardation	+	+	+	−
Chorioretinitis	++	−	++	+
Cataracts	−	++	−	−
Adenopathy	−	+	+	++
Dental defects	+	−	−	++

*– never or rare; + occurs; ++ has diagnostic importance.
Modified after C.J. Baker, MD, personal communication.

present at birth, but develop within the first few hours postpartum and last for 2 days. They are not always associated with thrombocytopenia.

- **Organomegaly.** Hepatomegaly and splenomegaly are the most common abnormalities. The liver is large, smooth, and nontender. Usually liver function tests are only mildly abnormal. The liver may remain enlarged up to 24 months, but usually returns to normal size in 12 months. Petechiae and splenomegaly may be the only clinical features of congenital CMV; splenomegaly tends to persist longer than hepatomegaly.
- **Jaundice.** Although jaundice is a common presentation, onset and severity are variable. Typically, the direct component of the bilirubin increases during the first week of life and can amount to 50% of the total bilirubin.
- **Microcephaly.** Microcephaly is a head circumference of <fifth percentile for gestational age. Intracranial calcifications can impair head growth and occasionally causes aqueductal stenosis and hydrocephalus. Although calcifications can occur anywhere in the brain, a periventricular location is typical (Fig. 6–1). Cerebral calcifications are a bad prognostic sign for neurodevelopmental outcome.
- **Ocular defects.** The principal ocular manifestations of CMV infections are chorioretinitis and optic atrophy. The chorioretinitis of CMV and toxoplasmosis are indistinguishable. Both produce central retinal lesions that impair fixation and cause strabismus. However, in contrast to toxoplasmosis, CMV chorioretinitis is less likely to be progressive.
- **Intrauterine growth retardation (IUGR).** IUGR occurs in as many as half and prematurity in one third of infants with symptomatic congenital CMV infection.

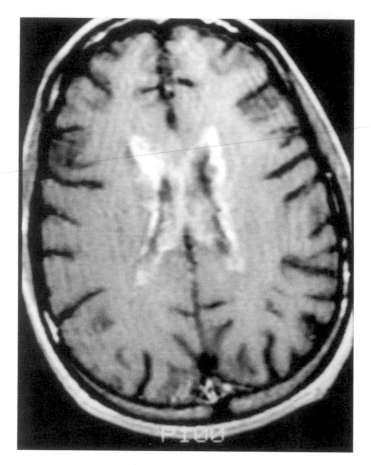

FIGURE 6–1   Human cytomegalovirus ventriculitis. Axial gadolinium-enhanced T1W-MRI showing contrast enhancement of ependyma of lateral ventricles. (Courtesy of J. Healy.)

- **Dental defects.** Children with congenital CMV infection can have enamel defects that lead to severe dental caries later in life.
- **Hearing loss.** Sensorineural hearing loss, the most common long-term sequelae of congenital CMV infection, is the most common, nonhereditary cause of sensorineural hearing loss in the United States. It occurs in up to 60% of children with symptomatic CMV disease and occurs after asymptomatic infection as well.

Diagnosis

To confirm congenital CMV infection, virus must be isolated within the first 2–3 weeks of life. After that time, virus shedding no longer differentiates congenital from postnatal infection. CMV can be isolated from urine, pharynx, peripheral blood leukocytes, human milk, semen, cervical secretions, and other tissues and body fluids. Urine and saliva are preferred samples for congenital CMV infection, because of their viral content. For these samples, a shell vial technique using monoclonal antibodies to detect CMV early antigens in inoculated fibroblasts grown on cover slips after centrifugation is diagnostic. Detection of CMV DNA by PCR or in situ hybridization of tissues and fluids is available in specialized laboratories. Quantitative CMV antigen assays by detecting pp65 antigen in white blood cells or quantitative CMV PCR allows risk assessment and therapy monitoring in the immunocompromised host. A strongly positive result of a test for serum anti-CMV IgM antibody is suggestive during early infancy, but IgM antibody assays are frequently false-positive or negative and not diagnostic by themselves. Computerized tomography (CT) of the brain shows periventricular calcifications.

Management

The antiviral agents currently approved for CMV treatment are ganciclovir (and its prodrug, valganciclovir), foscarnet, and cidofovir. The risk-benefit ratio of these agents in treating congenital CMV infection is uncertain. Limited data are available for ganciclovir. Ganciclovir is an acyclic analog of guanosine and inhibits CMV replication by inhibition of CMV DNA polymerase and DNA chain termination. Side effects include myelosuppression, renal and hepatic toxicity. CMV resistance may develop. A study by the National Institute of Allergy and Infectious Diseases Collaborative Antiviral Study Group (Kimberlin et al., 2003), found that starting ganciclovir therapy in newborns with symptomatic CMV infection involving the central nervous system prevents hearing deterioration at 6 months of life. Almost two-thirds of treated infants had significant neutropenia during therapy. Limiting the interpretation of study data was the large proportion of enrolled patients lost to follow-up. The benefits of any therapy are difficult to evaluate because brain damage is already considerable and perhaps complete at birth, while other organ derangements are usually self-limited.

Outcome

- **Symptomatic infection.** Death occurs in up to 30% of the most severely affected infants with multiorgan disease complicated by severe liver dysfunction, coagulopathy, bleeding and secondary sepsis. Newborns with symptoms of neurological dysfunction at birth usually have severe impairments (e.g. seizures, psychomotor retardation, cerebral palsy, and sensorineural hearing loss) later in life. Hearing loss and/or neurodevelopmental retardation occurs in 60% of patients with symptomatic congenital CMV disease. The presence of abnormalities on cranial CT scan within the first month of life is a good predictor that neurodevelopmental sequelae are to be expected.

- **Asymptomatic infection.** As many as 10 to 15% of infants with asymptomatic congenital CMV infection have or will develop neurological and/or developmental abnormalities which usually become apparent within the first 2 years of life. Of the children with asymptomatic congenital CMV infection, 7.2% develop sensorineural hearing loss (Fowler et al., 1997). In that study, progressions of hearing loss occurred in 50%, with the median age of 18 months at first progression. Delayed-onset sensorineural hearing loss was observed in 18.2% of asymptomatically CMV-infected children, with the median age of detection at 27 months.

Prevention

Because asymptomatic CMV shedding occurs in approximately 1% of all newborn infants, universal precautions and good hand hygiene are advisable, in particular after changing diapers. Universal screening is not a recommendation. A child with suspected or documented congenital CMV infection does not require special treatment or isolation. Some experts recommend serological testing of pregnant personnel prior to exposure to a child with known CMV excretion. Pregnant personnel require counseling about the potential risks of acquisition when caring for children of all ages. Compliance with good hand hygiene is required. The use of CMV antibody-negative donors, the freezing of red blood cells in glycerol before administration, removal of the buffy coat, and filtration to remove white blood cells has eliminated transmission of CMV by blood transfusion to newborn infants. Pasteurization or freezing of donated human milk can decrease the likelihood of CMV transmission. Because long-term sequelae are rare after CMV transmission through breast milk, many experts recommend no screening or treatment of breast milk if giving fresh breast milk is beneficial for the infant.

HERPES SIMPLEX VIRUS

Epidemiology

Herpes simplex virus (HSV) is a large DNA virus separated into two serotypes, HSV-1 and HSV-2. Traditionally, HSV-1 is associated with skin/eye/mouth infections ('above the belt') and HSV-2 with genital herpes. However, today HSV-1 causes at least 20% of genital herpes. The overall prevalence of genital herpes is increasing and approximately 25% of pregnant woman have serological evidence of past HSV-2 infection. The estimated rate of neonatal HSV disease is 1 in 3200 deliveries with 1500 cases occurring in the United States each year. Transmission of HSV to the newborn can occur in utero, peripartum, or postnatally (Arvin and Whitley, 2001). The majority of cases (~85%) are neonatal HSV-2 infections acquired during the time of delivery. Intrauterine infections are rare (<5% of infected infants or 1 in 300,000 pregnancies) and postnatal infections account for approximately 10% of infected infants. The highest risk for perinatal transmission occurs, when a mother with no prior HSV-1 or HSV-2 antibodies acquires either virus in the genital tract within 2 weeks prior to delivery (first-episode primary infection) (Kimberlin, 2004). Since cross-reactivity of antibodies exists, prior infection with HSV-1 offers some protection (first-episode nonprimary infection), which may explain the relative low rate of neonatal HSV disease despite the high prevalence of genital herpes. Postnatal transmission can occur with HSV-1 through mouth or hand by the mother or other caregiver. Characteristics of HSV, an *alpha herpesvirus*, are neurovirulence and the capacity for latency. During the first episode infection, which is commonly asymptomatic, HSV infects sensory nerve endings in skin or mucosal surfaces and transports via the nerve to the dorsal root ganglia. From the ganglia, it can reactivate, leading to shedding of infectious virus. Peripartum or postnatal HSV infections are classified as skin/eye/mouth disease (~45%), HSV encephalitis (~30%), or disseminated disease (~25%). All three types are potentially life threatening and can result in severe neurological sequelae.

Clinical Features

Intrauterine Infection

Skin vesicles and scarring, microphthalmos, chorioretinitis, retinal dysplasia, microcephaly or hydranencephaly evident shortly after birth suggest intrauterine HSV infection.

Skin/Eye/Mouth Disease

HSV skin/eye/mouth infection typically presents between 7 and 10 days as discrete 1–2 mm skin vesicles on erythematous base; crops of vesicles also occur. Eye disease appears as keratoconjunctivitis that can evolve into cataracts. Without treatment, approximately 70% of infants with skin/eye/mouth disease will develop disseminated HSV disease or HSV encephalitis. Severe neurological-sequelae develop in up to 10% of patients, despite antiviral treatment.

HSV Encephalitis

Most commonly, HSV encephalitis presents between 16–19 days postpartum, but sometimes as late as 4–6 weeks. Clinical features of HSV encephalitis are nonspecific and include seizures, lethargy, irritability, tremor, poor feeding, temperature instability, bulging fontanelle, and pyramidal tract signs. Between 60 and 70% of infants with HSV encephalitis have associated skin vesicles. According to a study by Whitley et al., the one-year mortality of treated HSV encephalitis was 14% and 56% of treated patients had neurological impairment (Whitley et al., 1991). Neurological sequelae include psychomotor retardation, often associated with microcephaly, or learning disability, hydranencephaly, porencephalic cysts, spasticity, and blindness.

Disseminated Disease

The onset of illness occurs usually between 10–12 days postpartum and clinical symptoms are indistinguishable from bacterial sepsis or neonatal enterovirus disease. Viremia accounts for the involvement of all organs, including CNS, respiratory tract, gastrointestinal tract (e.g. liver), kidneys, adrenals, spleen, pancreas, and heart. Possible symptoms are jaundice, respiratory distress, shock, and bleeding. Skin vesicles appear in 80% of affected children and encephalitis is present in 60–70%. In contrast to most cases of childhood HSV encephalitis, in congenital HSV, the virus enters the CNS via the bloodstream. This different route of viral spreading may explain the shorter incubation time and higher mortality of 60%, despite treatment. Neurological impairment occurs in 44% of survivors. Prematurity, coagulopathy and HSV pneumonitis indicate a poor prognosis.

Diagnosis

HSV grows well in tissue culture within 1–3 days. HSV isolation is by swabs from the base of skin vesicles, the mouth or nasopharynx, conjunctivae, urine, blood, stool or rectum, and CSF. Positive cultures after 48 hours of life suggest infection rather than colonization. HSV typing is of prognostic and epidemiologic interest. Polymerase chain reaction (PCR) detects HSV DNA and is of particular value for evaluating CSF, as cultures are frequently negative. In all cases of neonatal HSV disease, a diagnostic workup must include an evaluation for electrolyte abnormalities, neutropenia, thrombocytopenia, bleeding diathesis, as well as liver, pulmonary, and CSF involvement. In case of HSV encephalitis, blood cells and progressive increase of protein concentration is common in the CSF examination. CT or MRI brain imaging is useful to assess extent of disease and for follow-up evaluations. Close developmental monitoring for several years is important in all cases of neonatal HSV infections.

Management

Acyclovir inhibits HSV DNA polymerase and is effective against actively replicating HSV. Intravenous acyclovir is the drug of choice for all forms of neonatal HSV disease. The dosage is 60 mg/kg per day divided in three doses, given intravenously for 14 days in skin/eye/mouth disease and for 21 days in disseminated disease and in encephalitis. All patients with CNS HSV involvement should undergo a repeat lumbar puncture at the end of intravenous acyclovir therapy to determine that the CSF is PCR negative and normalized. Therapy continues until the PCR is negative. The main adverse effect of acyclovir is neutropenia. Monitor neutrophil counts at least twice weekly throughout the course of acyclovir therapy. The dose of acyclovir can be lowered or granulocyte colony-stimulating factor administered, if the absolute neutrophil count remains below 500/μL for a prolonged period. Relapse of diseases of the skin, eyes, mouth, and CNS can occur after cessation of treatment. The optimal management of these recurrences is not yet established. Infants with ocular HSV involvement should receive a topical ophthalmic drug (1–2% trifluridine, 0.1% iododeoxyuridine, or 3% vidarabine) as well as parenteral antiviral therapy.

Prevention

Complicating neonatal HSV disease prevention is the absence of genital herpes in more than 75% of women who deliver an infant with HSV infection, and who have no history of past infection or exposure at the time of delivery. Routine genital HSV cultures in the last weeks of pregnancy fail to predict the risk of perinatal infection. However, the risk of neonatal transmission is about 50% in women with primary infection in the last 2 weeks before delivery. In women with HSV reactivation, the risk of transmission is less than 5%. Elective cesarean section is usually only recommended if the mother has clinical features of recurrent or primary genital herpes at the onset of labor and ruptured membranes less than 4–6 hours. Neonatal infection has occurred despite cesarean section and in the absence of genital lesions; a maternal history of genital HSV is not an indication for cesarean delivery. Safety and efficacy of maternal suppressive therapy with acyclovir or valacyclovir prior to onset of labor are not established. Vaccines to prevent genital herpes are highly desired and in development. Avoid scalp monitors in infants of women suspected of having active genital herpes infection. Infants with visible lesions or infants born to mothers with active HSV lesions require contact precautions. Avoid postnatal transmission of HSV through family or hospital personnel with orolabial or genital herpes by coverage of active lesions and strict hand hygiene. Persons with herpetic whitlow should not have contact to newborns.

VARICELLA-ZOSTER VIRUS

Epidemiology

Varicella-zoster virus (VZV) is a member of the herpesvirus family and the source for chickenpox (varicella) after primary infection and zoster (shingles) after virus reactivation. Chickenpox is less contagious than measles but more than mumps or rubella. Most cases of chickenpox occur in nonimmunized school age children during the winter and spring months (Gershon, 2001). Even prior to universal childhood immunization, primary varicella disease in pregnancy was rare with estimated 1 to 5 cases per 10,000 pregnancies or between 350 and 1750 cases predicted per year in the United States. Zoster in pregnancy was more common with 6000 cases annually. The incubation period for varicella is usually 14 to 16 days, but prolonged for as long as 30 days after use of varicella-zoster immune globulin (VZIG) and shortened in immunocompromised patients. The absolute risk for congenital varicella syndrome after primary maternal VZV infection is less than

2% (Harger et al., 2002; Pastuszak et al., 1994). Infants born during the maternal incubation period do not suffer from varicella unless exposed postnatally. Infants born to mothers that develop varicella from 5 days before to 2 days after delivery are at risk for severe hemorrhagic varicella disease, because of lack of maternal antibodies. In contrast, infants >28 weeks' gestational age and born 5 days after the mother developed varicella receive maternal antibodies transplacentally and usually develop only mild symptoms.

Clinical Features

The clinical features in the newborn depend on the time of maternal infection. Zoster is rare and indicates early in-utero infection with VZV. Neurological symptoms are usual in the *congenital varicella syndrome*, characterized by skin scars, hypoplastic limbs, and eye and brain damage. Ocular abnormalities occur in half of patients with congenital varicella syndrome. These include chorioretinitis, Horner's syndrome, anisocoria, microphthalmia, cataract, or nystagmus. Cerebral cortical atrophy, diffuse brain disease, or mental retardation occurs in 40% of patients with congenital varicella syndrome. Seizures or myoclonic jerks are common. The combination of sensory, motor, urinary tract, gastrointestinal and limb abnormalities indicate damage to the spinal cord and autonomic nervous system.

Diagnosis

VZV can be isolated by culture within 3 to 7 days from scrapings of a vesicle base during the first 3 to 4 days of the rash. Virus antigen or DNA can be demonstrated from skin lesions and respiratory secretions. Presence of specific fetal IgM or persistence of VZV antibodies beyond 8 months of age strongly suggests intrauterine infection. Serum varicella IgG antibody tests can determine the immune status in healthy hosts but lack sensitivity in immunocompromised patients.

Management

Although safety and efficacy have not been established, acyclovir may be considered in pregnant woman and neonates with severe varicella disease. Dosages between 40 and 400 mg/kg/day of IV acyclovir have been proposed for severe varicella in the neonate.

Prevention

VZIG is prepared from donors with high antibody titers to VZV and can effectively modify varicella disease if given within 96 hours after exposure. Unfortunately, VZIG may no longer be available in the near future. The dose for neonates is usually one vial (1.25 mL) containing 125U by intramuscular injection to newborns whose mother had onset of chickenpox within 5 days before delivery or within 48 h after delivery. VZIG is not indicated if the mother has zoster or for healthy term infants exposed postnatally to varicella, including infants whose mother's rash developed more than 48 hours after delivery. However, some advise use of VZIG for any exposed susceptible newborn who has severe skin disease. In cases of significant exposure, give VZIG to hospitalized premature infants (28 weeks of gestation) whose mother lacks a reliable history of chickenpox or serological evidence of protection against varicella and to all hospitalized premature infants (<28 weeks of gestation or 1000 g birth weight), regardless of maternal history of varicella or varicella-zoster virus serostatus. Airborne and contact precautions are recommended for neonates born to mothers with active varicella and, if still hospitalized, should be continued until 21 days of age or 28 days of age if they received VZIG. Infants with active congenital varicella should be isolated together with their mothers. Patients with chickenpox are considered noninfectious when no new vesicles have appeared for 72 hours and all lesions have crusted.

RUBELLA

The rubella virus is a small, enveloped RNA virus with worldwide distribution and is responsible for an endemic mild exanthematous disease of childhood (German measles). Major epidemics, in which significant numbers of adults are exposed and infected, had occurred every 9 to 10 years in both the United States and the United Kingdom (Cooper et al., 2001). However, the incidence of rubella embryopathy in the United States had steadily declined with introduction of the rubella vaccine. The syndrome of congenital rubella as originally described was a triad of cataract, deafness, and congenital heart disease.

Epidemiology

Humans are the only known host for rubella virus. Transmission of postnatal rubella is primarily through direct or droplet contact from nasopharyngeal secretions. Highest risk of transmission is from five days before to six days after onset of the rash. Usually wild-type infection confers long-term immunity but reinfection may cause congenital rubella. Epidemics occurred in six to nine-year cycles prior to the vaccine era. The incidence of rubella in the United States has almost disappeared since. However, recent serological surveys indicate that approximately 10% of adults are nonimmune, most of which are foreign-born (Centers for Disease Control and Prevention (CDC), 2005). Gestational age at the time of maternal infection is the most important determinant of intrauterine transmission and fetal damage. In postnatal infection, the upper respiratory tract is the portal of viral entry. Following an incubation period of 9 to 11 days, an asymptomatic viremia occurs with lymphadenopathy as the only finding. Malaise, fever, and rash are typically so mild that almost one-half of mothers with definite intrauterine infection of their fetuses have no recollection of an antepartum illness. The maternal infection is self-limited, and symptoms ordinarily last no longer than one week. It is during the time of maternal viremia that the placenta and the fetus are infected. Congenital defects occur with first trimester infection in up to 85% of children. One large study that followed over a 1000 women with confirmed rubella infection at different stages of pregnancy reported congenital infection in more than 80% after infection during the first 12 weeks of pregnancy, 54% at 13–14 weeks, and 25% at the end of the second trimester (Miller et al., 1982). Maternal infection near term (>28 weeks) resulted again in higher transmission rates, suggesting that the placental barrier is relatively ineffective towards the end of pregnancy. The occurrence of congenital defects is as high as 85% if infection occurs during the first four weeks of gestation, 20% to 30% during the second month, and 5% during the third or fourth month. No defects occur when maternal infection is after 20 weeks. Infected infants can shed virus in nasopharyngeal secretions and the urine for several years.

Clinical Features

Clinical manifestations of congenital rubella can range from miscarriage to asymptomatic infection. Silent infections of the infant are more common. Up to 90% of infected infants appear healthy at birth. Because congenital rubella is a chronic infection, asymptomatic children require follow-up study. About 71% of these infants develop manifestations within 5 years. Table 6–1 lists the clinical manifestations of symptomatic congenital infection. Hepatosplenomegaly, jaundice, thrombocytopenia, myocarditis, cloudy cornea, and radiolucencies of long bones are self-limited, lasting days to weeks. Defects of the cardiovascular system, eye, CNS, and the genitourinary tract are often permanent. Sensorineural hearing loss occurs in more than 80% of infected infants. More than 50% of children infected in the first two months of gestation present with congenital heart disease, such as patent ductus arteriosus, pulmonary artery stenosis, and pulmonary vascular stenosis. Stenosis of other blood vessels can result in morbidity at later ages. The most common ocular finding is 'salt and pepper' retinopathy after disturbed growth of the pigmentary layer of the retina. Cataracts are present in approximately 33% and meningoencephalitis in 10 to 20% of newborns.

Diagnosis

Accurate counseling requires confirmation of rubella infection in the exposed pregnant woman. Documenting rubella-specific IgM antibody and a fourfold or greater rise in rubella-specific IgG documents the diagnosis. The 2003 Red Book states that the presence of rubella-specific IgG antibody at the time of exposure indicates immunity (Committee on Infectious Diseases, 2003). If antibody is not detectable, obtain a second blood specimen 2 to 3 weeks later and test it concurrently with the first specimen. If the second test result is negative, another blood specimen obtained 6 weeks after exposure is tested concurrently with the first specimen; a negative test result in both specimens indicates that infection has not occurred, and a positive test result in the second or third specimen but not the first (seroconversion) indicates recent infection. Children with suspected congenital rubella require attempts at viral isolation from the posterior pharynx, conjunctivae, CSF, and urine. Congenital rubella syndrome is suspect whenever there is a history of either maternal exposure or infection, or both, or if the child has IUGR associated with cataracts and congenital heart disease. Examination of the CSF may increase the index of suspicion for intrauterine infection. The protein content of the CSF is high in most newborns with rubella encephalitis, but it returns to normal after 3 months. In some, the protein concentration continues to increase after birth and remains elevated late into infancy. Virus isolation and the demonstration of IgM-specific antibody are most likely to be successful during the first months postpartum.

Management

All symptomatic or asymptomatic newborns with suspected congenital rubella should have a pediatric, neurological, cardiac, ophthalmologic, and audiological evaluation, including a complete blood count, CSF analysis, and radiographic bone studies. Long-term follow-up is crucial. Specific treatment is not available that can modify the course of rubella infection in the fetus or the newborn.

Outcome

Endocrinopathies, deafness, vision impairment, cardiovascular disease, and mental retardation adversely affect outcome. Progressive rubella panencephalitis is a late CNS manifestation, which is usually fatal.

Prevention

Children with proven or suspected congenital rubella require contact isolation until they are at least 1 year of age, unless repeated nasopharyngeal and urine culture results after 3 months of age repeatedly are negative for rubella virus.

Initial rubella immunization is at 12 to 15 months of age with a second dose at school entry at 4 to 6 years. Postpubertal females should not become pregnant for 28 days after receiving the vaccine, but inadvertent administration is not an indication for pregnancy termination. Immunize susceptible pregnant women during the immediate postpartum period before discharge. Breastfeeding is not a contraindication to immunization despite identification of vaccine virus in breast milk. All birth defects suspected secondary to rubella infection require a report to the Centers for Disease Control and Prevention through local or state health departments.

ENTEROVIRUS

Epidemiology

Enteroviruses are members of the picornavirus family and include coxsackieviruses A and B, echoviruses, polioviruses, and the newer enteroviruses identified by number. These single-stranded RNA viruses lack a lipid envelope, which results in relatively high resistance to environmental factors and alcohol. Since wild-type poliovirus is almost extinct, rare reports of neonatal disease are predominantly vaccine-associated. Therefore, this discussion focuses on nonpolio enteroviruses. Maternal infections with enteroviruses peak during summer and fall months in temperate climates and transmission to the neonate may occur during passage through the birth canal. Postpartum infection occurs by human contact directly and indirectly by fecal–oral route and respiratory secretions. The incubation period is short, 3–6 days, and nursery outbreaks are frequent.

Clinical features

Enteroviruses cause a variety of clinical symptoms, ranging from asymptomatic infection to a sepsis-like illness with liver failure (Cherry, 2001). Aseptic meningitis, encephalitis, and paralytic syndromes are clinical syndromes associated with enterovirus infections. Neonatal disease may also involve the lung, liver, and heart. The most severe neonatal disease is in preterm male infants with maternal illness within the 2 weeks prior to delivery. Specific enteroviruses are associated with particular diseases. Coxsackieviruses B1 through B5 and many echoviruses such as echovirus 9 and 11 are common causes of neonatal aseptic meningitis and meningoencephalitis. Enterovirus 71 is associated with brainstem encephalitis and polio-like paralysis. Echovirus 11 causes severe neonatal infections resembling neonatal sepsis. The clinical features of enterovirus meningitis or encephalitis include fever, lethargy, poor feeding, and irritability. Depending on the type of enterovirus and the severity of disease, other findings may include vomiting, diarrhea, rash, seizures, apnea, shock, thrombocytopenia, hepatomegaly, myocardial dysfunction and disseminated intravascular coagulation.

Diagnosis

Neonatal enterovirus disease resembles bacterial sepsis and herpes simplex virus disease. Important diagnostic factors are season of the year, geographic location, exposure, incubation period, and clinical symptoms. An important clue is a history of maternal illness consistent with enterovirus disease 1 to 3 weeks prior to delivery. CSF findings in enterovirus meningitis and meningoencephalitis are variable and can be similar to bacterial disease. For instance, hypoglycorrhachia occurs in 10% of newborns with enteroviral meningitis. Most enteroviruses can be isolated within 3 to 7 days from nose, throat, blood, urine, stool, and CSF. Swabs require transport media and then kept at 4°C until processing. Suckling mouse inoculation, which is not a routine procedure, is required for recovery of certain group-A coxsackievirus serotypes. Rapid virus identification by PCR is more sensitive than culture and equally specific. PCR identifies some enteroviruses from CSF, blood, urine, respiratory secretions, and tissue. Serology may be useful to determine specific enterovirus serotypes by collecting initial and convalescent titers.

Management

Management is predominantly supportive. Intravenous immunoglobulin is used but clinical efficacy not established. Preliminary studies suggest a clinical benefit for *pleconaril*, a relatively novel broad-spectrum anti-picornaviral agent. Pleconaril is orally bioavailable and concentrates within the central nervous system. Unfortunately, it is currently not available since it failed FDA approval as rhinovirus treatment. Enterovirus-infected infants require contact precautions for the duration of hospitalization, with particular attention to hand hygiene, especially after diaper changing.

LYMPHOCYTIC CHORIOMENINGITIS VIRUS

Epidemiology

Human infection with lymphocytic choriomeningitis virus (LCMV) occurs after contact with rodents such as mice, rats, hamsters and guinea pigs (Arvin and Maldonado, 2001). Mice and hamsters infected with LCMV remain asymptomatic but shed the virus in feces and urine for months. Human infection is by aerosol or ingestion of dust or food contaminated by rodent body fluids.

Clinical Features

About 75% of infected persons develop flu-like symptoms such as fever, headache, nausea, and myalgia lasting 5 to 15 days. A biphasic course and neurological complications such as aseptic meningitis or encephalitis are common. Infection during pregnancy can result in abortion, intrauterine infection, and perinatal infections. Spontaneous abortions occurred one month after symptomatic maternal infection as late as 32 gestational weeks. The most commonly described congenital anomalies are chorioretinopathy, intracranial calcifications, macrocephaly, and microcephaly (Barton and Mets, 2002). LCMV is a common cause of hydrocephalus. Up to one-third of newborns with hydrocephalus have positive serology to LCMV. In one study, almost 90% of children with serologically confirmed perinatal infection with LCMV had hydrocephalus (Sheinbergas, 1976). Almost 40% had hydrocephalus at birth; the remainder developed it over the first 3 months of age. Blindness and psychomotor retardation are potential long-term complications.

Diagnosis

Congenital LCMV may be difficult to differentiate clinically from congenital infection with cytomegalovirus, rubella virus, or toxoplasmosis. Viral culture of blood, CSF, and urine or serological studies confirms the diagnosis. Immunofluorescent antibody tests or enzyme-linked immunosorbent assays are currently available for serum and CSF. Polymerase chain reaction for detection of LCMV RNA may be available in the near future.

Prevention

Since specific antiviral therapy for LCMV is not established, pregnant women should avoid contact with rodents and their excretions. These recommendations apply to pet hamsters and laboratory animals, unless the animals are free of LCMV.

HUMAN IMMUNODEFICIENCY VIRUS TYPE 1

Epidemiology

Human immunodeficiency virus type 1 (HIV-1) is an enveloped retrovirus responsible for the vast majority of acquired immunodeficiency syndrome (AIDS) in the northern hemisphere. Approximately 1% of all reported AIDS cases in the United States are children. Acquisition of more than 90% of HIV-1 infections in children is from their mothers. The risk of infection for an infant born to an HIV-positive mother is between 13 and 39% if the mother did not receive any intervention during pregnancy and delivery. However, this number is highly dependent on the viral load and immune status of the mother, as well as events during labor and delivery. HIV transmission in HIV-infected mothers that do not breast-feed is approximately 30% in utero with the remainder during birth. HIV-1 is demonstrable in more than 70% of breast milk samples and contributes to infection in countries where no alternative to breast-feeding exists. The median age of onset of symptoms is approximately 12 to 18 months for untreated infants, but some children remain asymptomatic for many years. Serological response to HIV is evident 6 to 12 weeks after infection.

Clinical Features

The 2003 Red Book (Committee on Infectious Diseases, 2003) and the websites of the Centers for Disease Control and Prevention (www.cdc.gov/hiv/pubs.htm) list the clinical categories for children younger than 13 years of age with HIV infection and the pediatric HIV classification. The CNS manifestations of HIV disease in infants and children are separable into acute infectious complications (e.g. bacterial meningitis, CMV retinitis, *Toxoplasma gondii* encephalitis, and cryptococcosis) and chronic complications, such as progressive multifocal leukoencephalopathy, CNS malignancies, and much more commonly HIV encephalopathy. In a multicenter epidemiologic study in the United States (Lobato et al., 1995), HIV encephalopathy was diagnosed in 178 (23%) of 766 children with perinatally acquired AIDS. The median age at diagnosis of encephalopathy was 19 months and associated with severe morbidity evidenced by frequent hospitalizations, severe immunodeficiency, and short survival.

The clinical category of HIV encephalopathy is defined as either (1) failure to attain or loss of developmental milestones or loss of intellectual ability, verified by standard developmental scale or neuropsychologic tests; (2) impaired brain growth or acquired microcephaly demonstrated by head circumference measurements or brain atrophy demonstrated by computed tomography or magnetic resonance imaging (serial imaging required for children younger than 2 years of age); or (3) acquired symmetric motor deficit manifested by two or more of the following: paresis, pathologic reflexes, ataxia, or gait disturbance. Early HIV-1 infection increases a child's risk for poor neurodevelopmental functioning. A large multicenter prospective cohort study by Chase et al. analyzed cognitive and motor development during the first 30 months of life in 595 infants born to women infected with HIV-1 (Chase et al., 2000). The study showed that HIV-1 infection was significantly associated with increased risk for all outcome events related to abnormal mental and motor growth. Differences between the 114 infected and 481 uninfected infants were apparent by 4 months of age.

Outcome

The development of opportunistic infections, progressive neurological disease, and severe wasting, is associated with a poor prognosis. Other poor prognostic indicators are a viral load of more than 300,000 copies/mL, a decreased $CD4^+$ T-cell count, and symptoms during the first year of life. Median survival was nine years prior to the availability of highly active antiretroviral therapy (HAART). With earlier use of combination therapy, prognosis and survival rates have improved.

Diagnosis

HIV DNA PCR is the preferred method for the diagnosis of HIV infection in infants and children younger than 18 months of age. It is performed on peripheral blood mononuclear cells and highly sensitive and specific by two weeks of age. Approximately 30% of infants with HIV infection will have a positive DNA PCR assay result by 48 hours, 93% by 2 weeks, and almost all infants by 1 month of age. Positive test results need to be repeated. An infant can be considered not infected, when two HIV DNA PCR assays performed at or beyond one month of age, and a third performed on a sample obtained at four months of age or older, are negative. Alternatively, an infant with two negative HIV antibody tests obtained after six months of age and at an interval of at least one month also can be considered HIV-negative. Neuroimaging studies are useful for diagnosis.

Basal ganglia calcification and cerebral atrophy associated with acquired microcephaly strengthens the diagnosis of HIV-associated encephalopathy.

Management

The introduction of HAART prolongs survival and slows the course of illness. The management of HIV infection is complex and specialist consultation. Guidelines for the use of antiretroviral agents in pediatric HIV infection are updated frequently and available at www.aidsinfo.nih.gov.

Prevention

Frequently updated guidelines on the use of antiretroviral drugs in pregnant HIV-1-infected women and interventions to reduce perinatal HIV-1 transmission in the United States are available on-line at www.aidsinfo.nih.gov. If available, HIV-infected women receive antiretroviral therapy during pregnancy, labor, and delivery. All exposed newborn infants, recognized before 7 days of age, receive zidovudine (AZT) even if their mothers did not receive AZT. In addition, the American College of Obstetricians and Gynecologists recommends that HIV-infected pregnant women with viral loads of 1000/mL or greater should be counseled regarding the potential benefit of elective cesarean delivery. A potential transmission rate of 2% is achievable if mothers with detectable HIV viral load receive antiretroviral therapy and undergoes elective cesarean delivery before onset of labor and before rupture of membranes. Avoid breastfeeding if safe alternatives exist.

TOXOPLASMOSIS

Epidemiology

The protozoan *Toxoplasma gondii* (*T. gondii*) named after the North African rodent, the gondi (Remington et al., 2001). Three major forms of the organism infect humans: invasive tachyzoites, oocysts holding sporozoites, and tissue cysts containing bradyzoites. The cat is the only definite host who acquires *T. gondii* from prey and uncooked meat. Cats intermittently shed oocysts into the feces, which sporulate between 1 and 5 days and may inhabit warm, moist soil worldwide. Sporulated oocysts can infect humans by ingestion of food or water contaminated by soil or cat litter. In the United States, however, the most common cause of human infection with *T. gondii* appears to be consumption of raw or undercooked meat containing tissue cysts. After cellular immunity is established, the infection reaches a latent stage with viable cysts in multiple tissues. The incubation period for acquired infection ranges from 4 to 21 days.

Transmission to the fetus occurs after primary infection of the mother, after which trophozoites cause parasitemia and systemic infection. Approximately 85% of woman of childbearing age in the United States are susceptible to acute infection with *T. gondii*. The estimated incidence of congenital toxoplasmosis in the United States is 1 in 1000 to 1 in 10,000 live births, which would result in 400 to 4000 cases each year. The incidence of transmission is less than 2% with maternal infection in the first 10 weeks of gestation and rises near 80% when it occurs close to term. However, the later the infection occurs in the fetus, the less severe the disease. The highest risk for severe congenital toxoplasmosis with severe sequelae is close to 50% after infection in the first trimester, followed by 25% in the second and <3% in the third trimester.

Clinical Features

In the pregnant mother, primary infection with *T. gondii* is usually not recognized. The most common symptoms are lymphadenopathy and fever, occasionally resembling infectious mononucleosis (Table 6–1).

The clinical picture in the newborn can vary from normal appearance to hydrops fetalis. The triad of hydrocephalus, chorioretinitis, and intracranial calcifications strongly suggest congenital toxoplasmosis, but rarely occurs. CNS infection usually occurs in symptomatic neonates. Table 6–2 lists CNS manifestations. Other generalized symptoms of congenital toxoplasmosis include a maculopapular rash, generalized lymphadenopathy, hepatomegaly, splenomegaly, jaundice, and thrombocytopenia.

The most common manifestation of congenital toxoplasmosis is subclinical infection; such infants are often of lower birth weight and born prematurely. Persistent CSF abnormalities (lymphocytosis and elevated protein) and development of chorioretinitis in the second and third decade of life are the most frequent signs in subclinical congenital infection. Subclinical congenital infection is important to recognize since most develop adverse sequelae, which may improve after treatment.

TABLE 6–2　CNS symptoms of congenital toxoplasmosis

- Chorioretinitis
- Obstructive hydrocephalus
- Intracranial calcifications
- Abnormal spinal fluid
- Microcephalus
- Seizures
- Sensorineural hearing loss
- Visual impairment
- Spasticities and palsies
- Learning disabilities and mental retardation

Diagnosis

Establishing the diagnosis requires detection of the organism, by serology, or both. Several different serological methods are commercially available. Since the interpretation is difficult, presume that any patient with positive IgG and IgM titers were recently infected and require further testing in a reference laboratory. One reference laboratory in the United States, the Toxoplasma Serology Laboratory of the Palo Alto Medical Foundation Research Institute (TSL-PAMFRI), offers confirmatory serological and PCR testing and methods for isolation of the organism. In addition, medical consultants are available for interpretation of test results and advice on management of patients.

Prenatal diagnosis: When suspecting an acute *T. gondii* infection in a pregnant woman, the presence of positive or rising IgM and IgG titers confirms the prenatal diagnosis. Detection of *T. gondii* DNA in amniotic fluid by polymerase chain reaction (PCR) is less invasive and likely more sensitive than trying to isolate parasites from fetal blood or amniotic fluid. Serial fetal ultrasonographic examinations monitor for ventricular enlargement and other signs of fetal infection. Not all cases of congenital infection are detectable early and newborns at risk require close follow-up.

Postnatal diagnosis: Because of the variability in clinical expression of disease and the high rate of subclinical infection, the diagnosis of congenital toxoplasmosis relies, largely, on laboratory tests. Histology, serology, and isolation of *T. gondii* from body fluids or the placenta by animal and cell inoculation establishes the postnatal diagnosis of congenital toxoplasmosis. PCR has allowed detection of *T. gondii* DNA in brain tissue, cerebrospinal fluid (CSF), vitreous and aqueous fluid, bronchoalveolar lavage (BAL) fluid, urine, amniotic fluid, and peripheral blood. A detailed physical, neurological, and ophthalmological examination with auditory brain stem response measurement should be part of the evaluation. Further diagnostic testing includes a complete blood cell count with differential (eosinophilia is common in newborns with congenital toxoplasmosis), liver and kidney function testing, brain computed tomography scan (looking for calcifications and hydrocephalus), and CSF analysis. A very high concentration of protein (greater than 1 g/dL), producing a xanthochromic appearance, is unique for congenital toxoplasmosis.

Treatment

The lack of large randomized controlled trials complicates treatment recommendations. Spiramycin treatment of pregnant women with acute primary toxoplasmosis decreases transmission from 58% to 23% and should be started as soon as possible once the diagnosis of maternal infection is made (Desmonts and Couvreur, 1979; Daffos et al., 1988). Spiramycin is an investigational drug in the United States but obtainable from the manufacturer with authorization from the US Food and Drug Administration. With confirmed fetal infection after 17 weeks of gestation or if the mother acquires infection during the third trimester, consider therapy with pyrimethamine (Daraprim) plus sulfadiazine to decrease the severity of sequelae in the fetus. Administer folinic acid (leucovorin) with pyrimethamine and sulfadiazine to protect the bone marrow from the suppressive effects of pyrimethamine. Corticosteroids have been used for congenital toxoplasmosis when CSF protein is >1 g/dL and when chorioretinitis threatens vision. The optimal duration of therapy for congenital toxoplasmosis is unknown but often continued for 1 year. Because of the high likelihood of fetal damage, termination of pregnancy is frequently recommended if *T. gondii* infection is confirmed and infection is thought to have occurred at less than 16 weeks of gestation or if the fetus shows evidence of hydrocephalus.

Outcome

If untreated, early transmission (before 24 weeks' gestational age) results in severe congenital toxoplasmosis. Infection can be suppressed and outcome significantly improved by maternal treatment. A placebo-controlled trial is therefore unethical. Most infants infected in utero are born with no obvious signs of toxoplasmosis on routine newborn examination. Of these up to 80% will develop learning or visual disabilities and 40% neurological abnormalities later in life. CSF abnormalities do not correlate with the development of sequelae. The most common manifestation is chorioretinitis; Table 6–2 lists other CNS manifestations. Because of the risk for relapse, congenitally infected infants should have ophthalmological examinations in 3–4 month intervals until they can reliably report visual symptoms.

Prevention

Specific hygienic measures as listed in Table 6–3 are currently the only method for primary prevention. Many European countries perform universal toxoplasmosis screening during pregnancy. However, because of lower incidence in the United States, toxoplasmosis screening is currently only recommended for woman at high risk or with routine ultrasound findings consistent with fetal toxoplasmosis.

BACTERIAL MENINGITIS

Epidemiology

Bacterial meningitis is more common in the neonatal period than in any other time of life. Estimated incidence ranges from 0.25 to 1 case per 1000 live births. With advances in supportive care and antibiotics, there has been a fall in mortality from neonatal meningitis over the past few decades to about 10%. Despite this, the estimates of neurological sequelae from this infection have remained in the 20–58% range (Polin and Harris, 2001). The basis for classification of neonatal sepsis and meningitis are generally by the time of onset after birth. Presentations in the first 6 days of life are

TABLE 6–3   Prevention of toxoplasmosis in pregnant women

1. Cook food to a safe temperature (71.1°C [160°F]), and use a food thermometer to ensure that meat is cooked all the way through.
2. Peel or thoroughly wash fruits and vegetables before eating.
3. Wash cutting boards, dishes, counters, utensils, and hands with hot soapy water after they have been in contact with raw meat, poultry, or seafood, or with unwashed fruits or vegetables.
4. Pregnant women should wear gloves when they are gardening or touching soil or sand, because of the possible presence of cat feces. Afterwards, they should wash their hands thoroughly.
5. If possible, pregnant women should avoid changing cat litter pans. If no one else is available to change the cat litter, pregnant women should wear gloves for this task and then wash their hands thoroughly. The litter box should be changed daily, because *T. gondii* oocysts require more than 1 day to become infectious. Pregnant women should be encouraged to keep their cats inside and not to adopt or handle stray cats. Feed cats only canned or dried commercial cat food or well-cooked table food; they should never receive raw or undercooked meat.
6. Health education for women of childbearing age should include information about preventing *T. gondii* transmission from food and soil. At the first prenatal visit, health care providers should educate pregnant women about food hygiene and avoiding exposure to cat feces.
7. Health care providers who care for pregnant women should be educated about two potential problems associated with *T. gondii* serology tests: (1) no assay can determine precisely when initial *T. gondii* infection occurred; (2) in populations with a low incidence of *T. gondii* infection (e.g. U.S. population), a substantial proportion of positive IgM test results probably will be false positive.

Adapted from Preventing congenital toxoplasmosis. Centers for Disease Control and Prevention. MMWR Morb Mortal Wkly Rep 2000;49(RR-2):57–75.

referred to as early onset, although most early-onset sepsis occurs in the first 48 hours of life. Late-onset sepsis and meningitis occur after 7 days of life with a median age of 27 days. The most significant factors that predispose young infants to bacterial sepsis and meningitis are prematurity and low birth weight. Multiple studies have shown that the rate of meningitis is inversely proportional to birth weight. Other risk factors for early-onset sepsis and meningitis include prolonged (>18 hours) rupture of membranes, maternal chorioamnionitis, low socioeconomic status, male gender and need for invasive monitoring or resuscitation.

GROUP B STREPTOCOCCUS (GBS)

The species *Streptococcus agalactiae* is a beta-hemolytic, Gram-positive coccus, commonly referred to as Group B Streptococcus (GBS) by its Group B cell wall polysaccharide Lancefield classification. Previously an uncommon cause of human infection, GBS rather quickly became a leading cause of neo-natal sepsis and meningitis during the 1970s and has remained a major neonatal pathogen since that time. GBS colonizes roughly a quarter of women at the time of delivery and approximately 50% of colonized women transmit the organ-ism vertically. Additionally, GBS colonizes 5% of neonates whose mothers are culture-negative for GBS during their first 2 days of life (Edwards and Baker, 2001).

Neonatal GBS infection, similar to other causes of sepsis and meningitis, consists of patterns of disease specific to the age of the infant at onset. About 90% of early onset infections manifest by 48 hours of age but include all presentations in the first 6 days of life. Since the adoption of guidelines for intrapartum antibiotic prophylaxis in the mid 1990s, the overall attack rate for invasive neonatal GBS infection is about 0.6/1000 live births for early onset disease (Edwards and Baker, 2001). Meningitis is infrequent in early onset disease, present in 5–10% of cases. Late onset disease is infection presenting between 7 days and 3 months of age and has an incidence of roughly 0.2/1000. In late onset infection, meningitis is present in about 40% of cases. A third category, termed late, late onset, occurs after 3 months of age and primarily affects those babies born prematurely. Meningitis is infrequent in late, late onset infection. Five predominant GBS serotypes cause invasive neonatal infection, the frequency of each varying with the onset of disease. Across all three patterns of onset, serotype III is responsible for about 90% of cases of GBS meningitis.

GRAM-NEGATIVE BACILLI

Enteric Gram-negative rods are responsible for about a third of neonatal men-ingitis. In most published series, *E. coli* is second only to GBS in frequency, causing an estimated 15–20% of all cases (Klein, 2001). This occurs as both early and late onset disease. As in GBS, the distribution of *E. coli* isolates caus-ing meningitis is mainly a single serotype. The K1 polysaccharide capsular anti-gen is present in about 80% of *E. coli* isolates causing meningitis (Sarff et al., 1975). These strains are in the genital tract of mothers whose infants eventually infected; therefore, the transmission occurs during delivery. High rates of colo-nization with the K1 serotype occur in nursery staff, so postnatal acquisition in the nursery is also possible.

Other enteric Gram-negative bacilli, which are commensals of the human gastrointestinal or female genital tracts are also occasional causes of neonatal meningitis. *Klebsiella*, *Enterobacter*, *Citrobacter*, *Proteus* and *Serratia* species all appear in case series of meningitis in young infants at rates from <1% to almost 10% each (Klein, 2001). Three particular species, *Citrobacter koseri* (formerly *C. diversus*), *Serratia marcescens* and *Enterobacter sakazakii*, although rare, deserve special mention. These species have a strong association with cerebral abscess formation when causing meningitis in neonates. In meningitis caused by other bacteria, parenchymal brain abscesses are uncommon.

LISTERIA MONOCYTOGENES

Listeria monocytogenes is a motile, Gram-positive bacillus found in many environmental sources, including soil and organic matter. It is a significant cause of severe infections in animals, which in turn serve as the main source of colonization and infection of humans through ingestion of contaminated food products. Rates of lower gastrointestinal carriage in adults, including pregnant women, vary from 1% in hospitalized patients to 26% in household contacts of an infected patient. The majority of invasive human disease occurs in immuno-compromised adults. Neonatal infection occurs in the U.S. at an annual rate of 13/100,000 live births and accounts for about a third of all listeriosis. In times of food-borne outbreaks, neonates are disproportionally affected. As with other neonatal pathogens, early and late-onset patterns of disease are distinct. In *Listeria* infection manifesting prior to day 7 of life, meningitis occurs in 25% of patients. In late-onset disease, however, 95% of neonates have evidence of meningitis (Bortolussi and Schlech, 2001).

OTHER BACTERIA

Several bacteria, traditionally thought to affect only older children and adults, occur in neonates at a relatively low frequency. *Streptococcus pneumoniae*, *Haemophilus influenzae*, *Neisseria meningitidis*, and *Streptococcus pyogenes* (Group A) all occasionally colonize the female genital tract and present in neonates as early or late onset sepsis and meningitis. Group A Streptococcus (GAS) has been known for centuries as a cause of puerperal sepsis. Neonates acquire GAS by several routes: transplacental (from maternal bacteremia), intrapartum (from colonization/infection of the maternal genital tract), and post-partum (from contact with those with pharyngeal carriage or infection). GAS sepsis/meningitis is a rare, but frequently fatal condition in those neonates who do acquire the organism around the time of birth. As causes of meningitis in the U.S., *S. pneumoniae*, *H. influenzae* (mostly the nontypable variety) and *N. meningitidis* are as or more frequent in the first month of life than at any age beyond 2 years, according to a surveillance study done by the CDC in the 1980s (Klein, 2001). *Staphylococcus epidermidis* is the major cause of late onset sepsis in premature neonates, but infrequently causes meningitis. *Staphylococcus aureus*, *Salmonella* spp. and *Pseudomonas aeruginosa* are also uncommon causes reported in series of bacterial meningitis in neonates, as well.

Pathogenesis

Bacterial colonization of the baby usually occurs by acquisition of maternal genital flora. Colonization of the neonate's skin, eyes, mucous membranes, and umbilical cord occurs during vaginal birth, whereas babies born by cesarean section are relatively sterile in the first hours after birth. When rupture of membranes occurs prior to delivery, colonization and even infection of the fetus commonly occurs in utero. Although most neonates remain asymptomatically colonized, minor trauma to the skin or mucosa by invasive monitoring (e.g. with a scalp electrode) or devices used to assist delivery (e.g. forceps) and resuscitation (e.g. endotracheal intubation or suctioning) can serve as a portal of entry for colonizing organisms to cause infection. Similar infections occur in babies with intrinsically poor barrier integrity (e.g. premature infants).

Once bacteria gain access to the neonate's bloodstream, frequent absence of specific neutralizing antibody, immature function of phagocytes and immature inflammatory response to infection make newborns less likely to clear the infection. Hematogenous spread to the meninges is the primary mechanism of meningitis in neonates. Bacterial entry into the meninges occurs by passage through the blood–brain barrier of vascular endothelial cells or tight endothelial junctions in the choroid plexus and arachnoid membrane. Virulence factors in certain bacteria are known to aid in this attachment process, such as the expression of fimbriae in the K1 *E.coli* that bind cerebral endothelial glycoproteins. After entering the cerebrospinal fluid (CSF), bacteria are initially free to replicate in this relatively immunologically privileged site. However, bacteria soon die and release antigens such as lipopolysaccharides (LPS) and peptidoglycans that stimulate an inflammatory response. The cytokines (e.g. IL-1, TNF-a) and chemokines of this response attract leukocytes and aid in their attachment and penetration into the CSF.

Major pathological features include ventriculitis, cerebral edema, vasculitis, and infarction and periventricular leukomalacia. Brain injury caused by bacterial meningitis is multifactorial. Changes in cerebral blood flow, release of excitatory amino acids that lead to disrupted cellular electrolyte balances, and direct toxic effects of inflammatory cytokines and oxygen radicals all cause cell death in the brain and supporting tissue. Later sequelae of this damage include hydrocephalus, cystic encephalomalacia, venous thrombosis, subdural effusion, and hemorrhage. Cerebral abscesses are uncommon but occur with infections by *Citrobacter koseri* (formerly *C. diversus*) and *Enterobacter sakazakii* and may complicate meningitis from more common organisms (Willis and Robinson, 1988). Such abscesses are multiple, poorly encapsulated lesions that lead to necrosis and liquefaction of brain parenchyma.

Clinical Features

The signs of bacterial sepsis and meningitis in neonates are usually nonspecific and often subtle. Early onset sepsis, which includes meningitis in a minority of cases, may be apparent before delivery with signs of fetal distress, such as tachycardia. Upon delivery, term infants with low Apgar scores (e.g. <6 or 7) have been shown to be at higher risk for sepsis. In premature and low birth weight infants, Apgar scores have lower predictive value for sepsis, as these neonates are more likely to have low Apgars for other reasons. Fever (usually defined as temperature >38°C) is the only sign present in the majority of babies in series of neonatal meningitis, but occurred in only 61% of cases. Lethargy, anorexia or vomiting, and respiratory distress occur in about half of neonates with meningitis. Signs suggestive of the CNS as a focus of infection occur in the minority of cases: seizures in about 40%, irritability in 32%, bulging fontanelle in 28% and nuchal rigidity in only 15% (Klein, 2001). Focal neurological signs that occur but are uncommon include hemiparesis and abnormalities of cranial nerves VII, III and VI. Decreased urine output and hyponatremia may indicate the syndrome of inappropriate antidiuretic hormone secretion. Diabetes insipidus is a rare complication of meningitis.

Diagnosis

Lumbar puncture (LP) for examination and culture of CSF is the only reliable method of diagnosing meningitis. The indications for LP in neonates with suspected sepsis are not established. The relatively infrequent occurrence of bacterial meningitis in the setting of early-onset sepsis has led many pediatricians and neonatologists to defer LP until blood culture or another clinical specimen has confirmed bacterial sepsis. Since meningitis is present in 25% of neonates with bacteremia, a positive blood culture is an accepted indication for LP to guide therapeutic choices and prognosis. However, retrospective data shows that 15–50% of babies with culture-proven bacterial meningitis have concurrently negative blood cultures. Therefore, LP is an essential part of the initial evaluation of suspected sepsis (Wiswell et al., 1995; Stoll et al., 2004). Intrapartum maternal antibiotics can potentially sterilize the neonate's blood, further decreasing the negative predictive value of blood culture for meningitis. Conditions that would predispose to complications from LP, such as marked thrombocytopenia, coagulopathy or cardiopulmonary instability, are reasonable indications to defer examination of CSF.

Evaluation of CSF obtained from a neonate with suspected meningitis includes cell counts with leukocyte differential, glucose, protein, Gram stain and bacterial culture. Normal values for CSF leukocyte counts in neonates vary, but generally, normal ranges are from 0–22/mm^3 in term and 0–25/mm^3 in premature neonates. Additionally, many consider the presence of more than one neutrophil abnormal. Normal CSF glucose levels are 34–119 mg/dL (44–128% of serum glucose) for term and 24–63 mg/dL (55–105% of serum glucose) for preterm neonates. Normal CSF protein levels are 20–170 mg/dL for term and 65–150 mg/dL for preterm neonates. Absence of pleocytosis in cases of neonatal bacterial meningitis may occur when LP is early in the course of illness. However, this is exceptional; neonates with bacterial meningitis usually have hundreds to thousands of leukocytes per cubic millimeter of CSF. A 'bloody' tap cannot reliably exclude meningitis. Repeat of the procedure a day or two later can be valuable in such cases. Gram stain of CSF will reveal organisms in roughly 80% of cases of bacterial meningitis (Klein, 2001). Culture is the 'gold standard' for diagnosis, but can be negative in newborns exposed to antibiotics prior to LP, either in utero or postnatally.

Treatment

Rapidly administer empiric antibiotic therapy when suspecting sepsis or meningitis. Optimally, complete blood and CSF cultures prior to starting antibiotics, but never delay therapy for cultures. Initial therapy with intravenous ampicillin and gentamicin provides adequate coverage for GBS, *Listeria monocytogenes*, and many of the less frequent causes. If gram-negative bacilli are present in the CSF or highly suspected for other reasons (e.g. in the presence of cerebral abscesses), the addition of a third generation cephalosporin, such as cefotaxime, is suggested. It is important to note that cephalosporins have no appreciable activity versus *Listeria monocytogenes* and *Enterococcus* spp., which occasionally cause neonatal sepsis and meningitis. For this reason, ampicillin is preferred as part of the empiric regimen. Empiric therapy for the preterm neonate with late-onset sepsis should include vancomycin, as *Staphylococcus* spp., including coagulase-negative staphylococci, are important pathogens (although infrequent causes of meningitis) in this group of patients.

Positive culture results from CSF and/or blood are the basis for definitive therapy. Therapy for GBS meningitis should consist of intravenous aqueous penicillin G or ampicillin. The recommended doses of these agents for GBS meningitis are much higher than doses used for other infections. Penicillin doses are 250,000 to 450,000 U/kg/day divided into three doses for infants younger than a week old and 450,000 to 500,000 U/kg/day divided into 4 to 6 doses for older neonates. For ampicillin, the doses are 200–300 mg/kg/day divided into three doses if younger than a week and 300 mg/kg/day divided into 4 to 6 doses for those older than a week. The addition of an aminoglycoside, such as gentamicin, provides synergy in vitro, but no clinical data exist to suggest the superiority of this combination. Many experts recommend the addition of gentamicin until documenting a sterile repeat CSF culture 24–48 hours after beginning therapy. Cefotaxime is active versus GBS and likely to be effective for treatment of GBS meningitis, although clinical data is limited. Total therapy of 14–21 days is optimal, but 14 days is sufficient in uncomplicated cases. Treat listeria meningitis with ampicillin and gentamicin for 14–21 days. Trimethoprim-sulfamethoxazole is the alternative agent for patients with Listeria who are allergic to or intolerant of ampicillin. Treatment of gram-negative bacillary meningitis usually consists of dual therapy with either ampicillin or cefotaxime and an aminoglycoside for 21 days or 14 days after achieving sterilization of CSF. The exception to this generalization is *Pseudomonas*, which requires therapy with a beta-lactam agent with anti-pseudomonal spectrum such as ceftazidime. Definitive therapy for other less common causes of neonatal meningitis generally requires only monotherapy. Base the choice of agent on the susceptibility pattern of the individual isolate and the penetration of the antibiotic into the CSF of neonates. Intraventricular instillation of antibiotics, such as gentamicin, is associated with increased mortality and contraindicated.

Outcome

Case-fatality rates for neonatal meningitis are 20–25%, with term neonates faring better than premature babies (Klein, 2001). Up to half of survivors develop significant long-term neurological sequelae, including hearing impairment, hydrocephalus, seizure disorders, cerebral palsy, and mental retardation. Outcome data specific to GBS and for Gram-negative bacillary meningitis is available. In a few studies with long-term follow-up, GBS meningitis was associated with some abnormality in 40–50% and Gram-negative meningitis with 56% abnormal in follow-up of survivors. Poor outcomes with GBS are predictable by comatose states at presentation, peripheral WBC count <5000/mm^3, absolute neutrophil count <1000/mm^3, and CSF protein >300 mg/dL. For Gram-negative meningitis, thrombocytopenia, CSF WBC >2000/mm^3, CSF protein >200 mg/dL, CSF/blood glucose ratio <0.5, and positive CSF cultures >48 hours were factors associated with poor outcomes. About half of neonates with brain abscesses die, and the majority of survivors have seizures and mental retardation.

Prevention

Only in GBS disease is neonatal sepsis and meningitis proven to be preventable. Intrapartum antibiotic prophylaxis instituted in the mid-1990s reduced the rates of early-onset GBS disease by 65% but has not had a clear effect on late-onset disease (Edwards and Baker, 2001). Universal screening of women in the third trimester with a recto-vaginal culture for GBS is the most effective method of determining which women should receive prophylactic antibiotics during labor. A risk-based approach, without culture screening, was once an acceptable alternative to determine indication for prophylaxis; however, the risk-based approach misses a substantial number of early-onset GBS cases as compared to culture-based screening. Give intrapartum penicillin or ampicillin to culture-positive women in labor, beginning at least 4 hours prior to delivery, to prevent early-onset neonatal disease. Studies of vaccines for protection against GBS show that capsular polysaccharide type-specific IgG is protective from GBS infection. Efforts to develop a maternal vaccine to protect infants from GBS disease have evolved from early trials that show the poor immunogenicity of GBS polysaccharide antigen vaccine to more recent efforts studying protein conjugated polysaccharide vaccines. At present, no approved GBS vaccines are available.

Recommendations for prevention of Listeria infections include that pregnant women should avoid eating soft cheeses, unpasteurized dairy products and refrigerated meat spreads (such as pâtés), thoroughly heat ready-to-eat foods (e.g. hot dogs) and consider avoiding foods that come from delicatessen counters, such as cold cuts of meat.

CANDIDA INFECTION OF THE CNS

Epidemiology

Invasive infection with the yeast, *Candida* spp., is common in hospitalized neonates. *Candida* is the second most common cause of late-onset sepsis in very low birth weight babies, including an estimated 4% to 15% attack rate in extremely low birth weight babies (Benjamin et al., 2003a). Risk factors for candidemia in neonates include gestational age less than 32 weeks, prior use of intralipid, parenteral nutrition, cephalosporin or carbapenem antibiotics and H_2 blocking medications (Saiman et al., 2000 and Benjamin et al., 2003a). The attributed mortality from invasive candidiasis in neonates is 38% (Benjamin et al., 2003a). Neonatal candidemia commonly leads to disseminated foci of infection, and *Candida* infection of the central nervous system in neonates occurs most commonly as meningitis resulting from this hematogenous spread. CNS candidal infections also occur infrequently as complications of neurosurgical procedures or instrumentation by spread from contiguous skin. Although reported data on complications of candidemia consist mostly of relatively small case series, a thorough meta-analysis found the median reported prevalence of meningitis to be 15% in neonatal *Candida* bloodstream infections (Benjamin et al., 2003b). A large, single-center review reported meningitis in 25% of neonates with systemic candidiasis (Fernandez et al., 2000).

Candida albicans remains the most common species seen in invasive infections, although *C. parapsilosis* accounts for a greater proportion of neonatal cases in comparison to other age groups. Animal models suggest that *C. albicans* has the most invasive potential of *Candida* spp., and in neonates, clinical data suggests a higher prevalence of meningitis in those whose infecting species was *C. albicans*. *C. tropicalis*, *C. lusitaniae* and *C. glabrata* also cause neonatal meningitis.

Clinical Features

Unfortunately, no clinical features reliably distinguish candidal from bacterial meningitis or from non-CNS candidiasis. Common nonspecific findings include feeding intolerance, respiratory distress, increased apnea and bradycardia, hypotension, temperature instability, mottling, and metabolic acidosis. As with neonatal bacterial meningitis, signs such as nuchal rigidity or fullness of the fontanelle have poor negative predictive value.

Diagnosis

Given the relatively high incidence of meningitis in neonates with systemic candidiasis, lumbar puncture is indicated when any infection with *Candida* spp. is present or suspected. The principles of evaluation and interpretation of CSF discussed earlier in the bacterial meningitis section apply to neonates suspected of having Candida meningitis, as well. The CSF findings of neonates with culture-proven meningitis are quite variable. In the largest series of patients, those with definite meningitis had an overall mean number of CSF WBCs = 215/mm^3 and a median of 52.5/mm^3 (Fernandez et al., 2000). Perhaps the most striking finding in that series was that the minority with definite candidal meningitis had a CSF pleocytosis, and of those, mononuclear cells (rather than neutrophils) usually predominated. Hypoglycorrhachia occurred in about a quarter of patients (mean CSF glucose = 95 mg/dL), and the mean CSF protein was 214 mg/dL. Interestingly, Gram-staining of CSF was uniformly negative. Culture of CSF is generally the basis by which to make the diagnosis. However, in patients with candidemia who have received antifungal therapy prior to LP, abnormal CSF findings are putative evidence of candidal meningitis, even if cultures do not grow the organism.

Because candidal meningitis is part of a disseminated infection, other potential sites of infection require evaluation. Obtain blood cultures at the beginning of the evaluation and then repeat daily until cultures are negative. Infections of the kidneys and urinary tract are frequent in neonates. Urine culture and renal ultrasound should be routine. Other occasional infections that result from candidemia are endocarditis and endophthalmitis, each occurring in 5% or less of babies (Benjamin et al., 2003b). Echocardiogram and slit-lamp examination are routine but the optimal timing of such studies is unknown. Delaying eye and kidney examination until near the end of treatment may help to exclude lesions that become apparent late in the course. When using an agent with unproven site-specific efficacy or penetration (e.g. an echinocandin antifungal), evaluate for dissemination at initial diagnosis.

Treatment

Amphotericin B deoxycholate, a fungicidal agent that binds to fungal membrane ergosterol, is the treatment of choice for serious fungal infections in neonates. The recommended maximal dose of intravenous amphotericin B is 1 mg/kg/day, with a total cumulative dose of 25–30 mg/kg. Reported series of neonatal candidal meningitis demonstrate efficacy of amphotericin B in a retrospective, noncomparative fashion. Clinical experience with the drug over the past 50 years is considerable. However, little data is available on the pharmacokinetics and comparative efficacy of this agent in neonates. Some indication exists from limited data that its penetration into the CSF of neonates is significantly better than in adults, where only 2–4% of serum levels of amphotericin penetrate into the CSF (van den Anker et al., 1995). Nephrotoxicity is the commonest side effect of amphotericin B, although tolerance in neonates is better than in adults. The nephrotoxicity is generally reversible with discontinuation of the drug; but requires monitoring of serum creatinine, potassium, magnesium, calcium, and phosphorus. Lipid formulations of amphotericin B offer lower rates of nephrotoxicity in older patients; limited data fails to show this effect for neonates. Liposomal amphotericin B (Ambisome®) penetrates brain tissue better than other formulations of amphotericin B in animals, but no human data is available to corroborate this finding.

Flucytosine (5-FC) is fluorinated pyrimidine that disrupts fungal protein synthesis and DNA replication after incorporation into RNA. The rapid emergence of resistance when given as monotherapy requires concurrent use of amphotericin B. Due to the superior penetration into the CSF, some experts recommend 5-FC in combination with amphotericin B for the treatment of candidal meningitis. However, data in neonates comparing this combination to monotherapy with amphotericin B is lacking. 5-FC is only available in an enteral preparation. The toxicity of 5-FC in adults is primarily myelosuppression, but the drug's safety has not been adequately studied to accurately describe side effects in neonates.

If 5-FC is given, serum concentration measurements are necessary since the toxicity in adults relates to levels greater than 100 µg/mL.

Fluconazole is a fungistatic triazole agent that inhibits synthesis of ergosterol for fungal cell membranes. Intravenous or oral administration achieves significant concentrations in most body fluids, including CSF. The toxicity profile is favorable relative to amphotericin B, with elevated hepatic enzymes being the most common side effect. As with other antifungal agents, however, clinical data in neonates is inadequate to make a strong recommendation for using fluconazole as primary therapy for candidal meningitis. Anecdotal reports of clinical failures of fluconazole for meningitis and uncertainty as to the optimal dosing in neonates underscore this concern. Another important consideration is that fluconazole resistance is common among non-albicans *Candida* spp., in particular *C. glabrata* and *C. krusei*. Susceptibility testing is required. A newer class of antifungal agents, the echinocandins, offers much promise in the treatment of Candida. Two agents, caspofungin and micafungin, are currently approved for use, although neither yet has an indication in neonates. These agents are fungicidal for *Candida* spp. and have no significant toxicity in older patients. However, data on neonates is lacking, and these drugs are therefore not used in neonatal candidal meningitis.

Outcome

Even with appropriate antifungal therapy, the case-fatality rate for neonates with candidal meningitis is at least 25% (Fernandez et al., 2000). This is due, in part, to the comorbidities that are nearly invariable in hospitalized neonates. As mentioned earlier, *C. albicans* appears to be the most pathogenic of *Candida* spp., and may lead to higher mortality rates in invasive infection in comparison to other species, such as *C. parapsilosis*. A significant proportion of survivors of neonatal candidal meningitis will have long-term sequelae such as psychomotor retardation, aqueductal stenosis and hydrocephalus.

Prevention

When possible, limiting use of intralipid, parenteral nutrition, cephalosporin and carbapenem antibiotics and H_2 blocking medications in premature neonates may aid in prevention of colonization and subsequent invasive infection with *Candida* spp. A number of well-done studies demonstrated that premature neonates given intravenous fluconazole on an intermittent schedule had lower rates of colonization with *Candida* spp. and fewer invasive candidal infections versus babies who received placebo (e.g. Kaufman et al., 2001). Due to unanswered questions regarding the effect on selection of resistant fungi and the safety of such a regimen in neonates, prophylactic fluconazole for infants at risk is not yet a universal practice in neonatal intensive care units but is standard in some institutions.

REFERENCES

Arvin AA and Maldonado YA. Lymphocytic choriomeningitis virus. In: JS Remington, JO Klein (eds). Infectious Diseases of the Fetus and Newborn Infant, 5th edn. Philadelphia: WB Saunders, 2001; pp. 860–862.

Arvin AA and Whitley RJ. Herpes simplex virus infections. In: JS Remington and JO Klein (eds). Infectious Diseases of the Fetus and Newborn Infant, 5th edn. Philadelphia: WB Saunders, 2001; pp. 425–446.

Barton LL and Mets MB. Congenital lymphocytic choriomeningitis virus infection: Decade of rediscovery. Clin Infect Dis 2002;33:370–374.

Benjamin DK Jr, DeLong ER, Steinbach WJ, et al. Empirical therapy for neonatal candidemia in very low birth weight infants. Pediatrics 2003a;112:543–547.

Benjamin DK, Poole C, Steinbach WJ, et al. Neonatal candidemia and end-organ damage: A critical appraisal of the literature using meta-analytic techniques. Pediatrics 2003b; 112:634–640.

Bortolussi R and Schlech WF. Listeriosis. In: JS Remington and JO Klein (eds). Infectious Diseases of the Fetus and Newborn Infant, 5th edn. Philadelphia: WB Saunders, 2001; pp. 1157–1177.

Centers for Disease Control and Prevention (CDC). Elimination of rubella and congenital rubella syndrome – United States, 1969–2004. MMWR Morb Mortal Wkly Rep 2005;54:279–282.

Chase C, Ware J, Hittelman J, et al. Early cognitive and motor development among infants born to women infected with human immunodeficiency virus. Women and Infants Transmission Study Group. Pediatrics 2000;106:E25.

Cherry JD. Enteroviruses. In: JS Remington, JO Klein (eds). Infectious Diseases of the Fetus and Newborn Infant, 5th edn. Philadelphia: WB Saunders, 2001; pp. 477–518.

Committee on Infectious Diseases. L Pickering, CJ Baker, GD Overturf and CG Prober (eds). The Red Book, 26th edn. American Academy of Pediatrics, 2003.

Cooper LZ and Alford CA. Rubella. In: JS Remington and JO Klein (eds). Infectious Diseases of the Fetus and Newborn Infant, 5th edn. Philadelphia: WB Saunders, 2001; pp. 347–388.

Daffos F, Forestier F, Capella-Pavlovsky M, et al. Prenatal management of 746 pregnancies at risk for congenital toxoplasmosis. N Engl J Med 1988;318:271–275.

Desmonts G and Couvreur J. Congenital toxoplasmosis: a prospective study of the offspring of 542 women with acquired toxoplasmosis during pregnancy: pathophysioloy of congenital disease. In: O Thalhammer, K Baumgartner and A Pollak (eds). Perinatal Medicine, Sixth European Congress, Vienna. Stuttgart: G Thieme, 1979; pp. 51–60.

Edwards MS and Baker CJ. Group B streptococcal infections. In: JS Remington and JO Klein (eds). Infectious Diseases of the Fetus and Newborn Infant, 5th edn. Philadelphia: WB Saunders, 2001; pp. 1091–1156.

Fernandez M, Moylett EH, Noyola DE and Baker CJ. Candidal meningitis in neonates: A 10-year review. Clin Infect Dis 2000;31:458–463.

Fowler KB, McCollister FP, Dahle AJ, et al. Progressive and fluctuating sensorineural hearing loss in children with asymptomatic congenital cytomegalovirus infection. J Pediatr 1997;130:624–630.

Frattarelli DA, Reed MD, Giacoia GP and Aranda JV. Antifungals in systemic neonatal candidiasis. Drugs 2004;64(9):949–968.

Gershon AA. Chickenpox, measles, mumps. In: JS Remington and JO Klein (eds). Infectious Diseases of the Fetus and Newborn Infant, 5th edn. Philadelphia: WB Saunders, 2001; pp. 683–708.

Harger JH, Ernest JM, Thurnau GR, et al. Frequency of congenital varicella syndrome in a prospective cohort of 347 pregnant women. Obstet Gynecol 2002;100:260–265.

Kaufman D, Boyle R, Hazen KC, et al. Fluconazole prophylaxis against fungal colonization and infection in preterm infants. N Engl J Med. 2001;345:1660–1666.

Kimberlin DW. Neonatal herpes simplex infection. Clin Microbiol Rev 2004;17:1–13.

Kimberlin DW, Lin CY, Sanchez PJ, et al. Effect of ganciclovir therapy on hearing in symptomatic congenital cytomegalovirus disease involving the central nervous system: A randomized, controlled trial. J Pediatr 2003;143:16–25.

Klein JO. Bacterial sepsis and meningitis. In: JS Remington and JO Klein (eds). Infectious Diseases of the Fetus and Newborn Infant, 5th edn. Philadelphia: WB Saunders, 2001; pp. 943–998.

Lobato MN, Caldwell MB, Ng P and Oxtoby MJ. Encephalopathy in children with perinatally acquired human immunodeficiency virus infection. Pediatric Spectrum of Disease Clinical Consortium. J Pediatr 1995;126:710–715.

Miller E, Cradock-Watson JE and Pollock TM. Consequences of confirmed maternal rubella at successive stages of pregnancy. Lancet 1982;2:781–784.

Moylett, EH. Neonatal Candida meningitis. Semin Pediatr Infect Dis 2003;14:115–122.

Pastuszak AL, Levy M, Schick B, et al. Outcome after maternal varicella infection in the first 20 weeks of pregnancy. N Engl J Med 1994;330:901–905.

Polin RA and Harris MC. Neonatal bacterial meningitis. Semin Neonatol 2001;6:157–172.

Remington JS, McLeod R, Thulliez P and Desmonts G. Toxoplasmosis. In: JS Remington and JO Klein (eds). Infectious Diseases of the Fetus and Newborn Infant, 5th edn. Philadelphia: WB Saunders, 2001; pp. 205–346.

Saiman L, Ludington E, Pfaller M, et al. Risk factors for candidemia in Neonatal Intensive Care Unit patients. Pediatr Infect Dis J 2000;19:319–324.

Sarff LD, McCracken GH Jr., Schiffer MS, et al. Epidemiology of *Escherichia coli* K1 in healthy and diseased newborns. Lancet 1975;1:1099–1104.

Schuchat A. Group B Streptococcus. Lancet 1999;353:51–56.

Schuchat A, Oxtoby M, Cochi S, et al. Population-based risk factors for neonatal group B streptococcal disease: results of a cohort study in metropolitan Atlanta. J Infect Dis 1990;162:672–677.

Shattuck KE and Chonmaitree T. The changing spectrum of neonatal meningitis over a fifteen year period. Clin Pediatr 1992;31:130–136.

Sheinbergas MM. Hydrocephalus due to prenatal infection with the lymphocytic choriomeningitis virus. Infection.1976;4:185–191.

Stagno S. Cytomegalovirus. In: JS Remington and JO Klein (eds). Infectious Diseases of the Fetus and Newborn Infant, 5th edn. Philadelphia: WB Saunders, 2001; pp. 389–424.

Stoll BJ, Hansen N, Fanaroff AA, et al. To tap or not to tap: High likelihood of meningitis without sepsis among very low birth weight infants. Pediatrics 2004;113:1181–1186.

van den Anker JN, van Popele NM and Sauer PJ. Antifungal agents in neonatal systemic candidiasis. Antimicrob Agents Chemother 1995;39:1391–1397.

Whitley R, Arvin A, Prober C, et al. A controlled trial comparing vidarabine with acyclovir in neonatal herpes simplex virus infection. N Engl J Med 1991;324:444–449.

Willis J and Robinson JE. Enterobacter sakazakii meningitis in neonates. Pediatr Inf Dis J 1988;7:196.

Wiswell TE, Baumgart S, Gannon CM and Spitzer AR. No lumbar puncture in the evaluation for early neonatal sepsis: will meningitis be missed? Pediatrics 1995;95:803–806.

7

Metabolic Disorders

Gerald M. Fenichel

All inborn errors of metabolism are present at birth, and most cause disturbances of the nervous system. This discussion is limited in scope to those conditions that ordinarily produce neurological dysfunction in the first month. Most result in a metabolic encephalopathy caused by enzyme deficiencies that impair substrate production and produce excessive intermediary metabolites and metabolites of alternative pathways. The nervous system can be injured by a direct toxic effect of the accumulated metabolites; deficiency of essential substrates; or by metabolic derangements such as severe acidosis, hyperammonemia, and hypoglycemia.

The initial clinical features of decreased states of consciousness and seizures often begin after dietary exposure to a substrate that the body fails to metabolize. Disturbances of amino acid metabolism are the main causes of metabolic encephalopathies in the newborn. Less frequent causes are lysosomal disorders that disturb glycogen metabolism and mitochondrial disorders. Peroxisomal disorders are symptomatic in the newborn but do not cause acute metabolic encephalopathies. Lysosomal disorders of mucopolysaccharide and lipid metabolism usually cause neurological dysfunction during infancy or childhood.

DISORDERS OF AMINO ACID METABOLISM

Disorders of amino acid metabolism usually present in the newborn following the initiation of protein feeding as an acute overwhelming disease characterized by acidosis, hypoglycemia, vomiting, and seizures. Important exceptions are those disorders that come to attention by virtue of newborn screening programs, rather than as disease states. Newborn screening programs differ from state-to-state and from country-to-country.

Hyperphenylalaninemia

Phenylketonuria

Pathophysiology   Phenylketonuria (PKU) is a disorder of phenylalanine metabolism secondary to a hepatic deficiency or total absence of the enzyme phenylalanine hydroxylase (PAH) (Ryan and Scriver, 2004). The PAH gene is located at chromosomal locus 12q24.1. Several different mutation may occur in the PAH gene and genotype does not closely predict phenotype (Scriver, 2002). Transmission of the defect is by autosomal-recessive inheritance. The prevalence of hyperphenylalinemia varies among different ethnic populations. Hydroxylation of phenylalanine to tyrosine is impaired causing excessive concentrations of phenylalanine to accumulate and penetrate all body tissues. The hydroxylase reaction, which is lacking in PKU, occurs only in the liver, but several other tissues (brain, liver, and kidney) are capable of transaminating phenylalanine to phenylpyruvic acid. Phenylacetic acid is the oxidation product of phenylpyruvic acid. The cause of the musty urine odor is the excretion of phenylpyruvic acid.

Hyperphenylalanemia affects myelination and cognitive development. Dysmyelination occurs even in children treated early and managed carefully. The most consistent pathological feature of PKU is microcephaly due to reduction in white matter volume. Structural changes within the white matter are age dependent. They begin as focal status spongiosis and progress to a generalized absence of myelination. Chemical analysis of cerebral lipids indicates an inadequate formation of myelin rather than active destruction of myelin.

The normal phenylalanine plasma concentration is 1.0–2.0 mg/dL. Neonatal screening programs detect children with hyperphenylalaninemia. Two-thirds of such children have classic phenylketonuria (PKU) caused by PAH deficiency, and most of the remainder has benign non-PKU hyperphenylalaninemia. Approximately 2% of patients with hyperphenylalaninemia have a defect in the generation or recycling of tetrahydrobiopterin, a necessary cofactor for the PAH reaction. An early, precise diagnosis is important because early dietary restriction of phenylalanine prevents the severe complications of classic PKU. Dietary restriction alone normalizes the plasma phenylalanine in newborns with the cofactor deficiency, but does not prevent neurological deterioration.

Clinical Features   In the absence of compulsory mass screening, classic PKU is not diagnosable in the newborn. Delay screening tests at least 24 hours after the first protein feeding. The most commonly used tests are the Guthrie test (a bacterial inhibition assay) and fluorometric determinations of phenylalanine. False-positive and false-negative results are possible. Infants with positive screening test results must have quantitative measurements of phenylalanine. Measures of tyrosine, urine pterins, and dihydropteridine reductase are required in any child with a positive screening test result. Disorders of tyrosine and pterin metabolism also cause elevations of phenylalanine concentrations. Table 7–1 lists the differential diagnosis of a positive neonatal screening test.

Untreated homozygotes, although normal at birth, show progressive developmental delay, which is not usually evident until 2 or 3 months of age. Mental

TABLE 7-1   Differential diagnosis of hyperphenylalaninemia

Classic phenylketonuria
Complete hydroxylase deficiency (zero to 6%)

Benign variants
Other
Partial hydroxylase deficiency (6% to 30%)
Phenylalanine transaminase deficiency
Transitory hydroxylase deficiency

Malignant variants
Dihydropteridine reductase deficiency
Tetrahydrobiopterin synthesis deficiency

Tyrosinemia
Transitory tyrosinemia
Tyrosinosis

Liver disease
Galactose-1-phosphate uridylyl transferase deficiency

---

retardation is inevitable in untreated infants with complete absence of PAH but is less constant among some of the variant forms. Two-thirds of children with PKU have blond hair and blue eyes, regardless of their parents' coloration, because of disturbances in pigment formation.

With the success achieved in treating newborns with PKU, homozygous females have married and borne children of their own. The heterozygote fetus of homozygote mothers develop in an abnormal metabolic milieu. Amino acids pass through the placenta freely and have a tendency to accumulate in the fetus, in which enzymes for metabolism are not yet mature. Infants born to mothers with hyperphenylalaninemia are at increased risk for microcephaly, mental retardation, and congenital malformations despite the fact that the infant's enzyme activity is half of normal. Damage to the fetus relates directly to the mother's phenylalanine plasma concentration. Even at maternal plasma phenylalanine concentrations of 2–6 mg/dL, 6% of infants are born with microcephaly and 4% with postnatal growth retardation. At plasma concentrations above 15 mg/dL, the risk is 85% for microcephaly, 51% for postnatal growth retardation, and 26% for intrauterine growth retardation. Hyperphenylalaninemic women must maintain nutritional therapy at least through their childbearing years.

Classic PKU occurs when PAH deficiency is 0–6% of normal. Serum phenylalanine levels are 20 mg/dL or greater, and serum tyrosine levels are less than 5 mg/dL. Plasma phenylalanine concentrations rise more rapidly in newborns fed cow's milk instead of nursing. Human breast milk is relatively low in phenylalanine content. Such individuals tolerate less than 250 to 350 mg of dietary phenylalanine per day to keep plasma concentrations at a level less than 300 μmol/L (5 mg/dL). Without dietary treatment, most individuals develop profound, irreversible mental retardation.

Individuals with moderate PKU tolerate 350–400 mg of dietary phenylalanine per day and those with mild PKU tolerate 400–600 mg of dietary phenylalanine per day. Children with mild PKU may not require dietary treatment. Phenylalanine concentrations less than 25 mg/dL with normal concentrations of tyrosine characterize benign variants of PKU. The *benign variants* are caused either by partial PAH deficiency or transitory hydroxylase deficiency. Screening detects these newborns.

The causes of *malignant hyperphenylalaninemia variants* are disorders in the metabolism of tetrahydrobiopterin, a cofactor for PAH, tyrosine hydroxylase, and tryptophan hydroxylase. They are responsible for 1–3% of cases of hyperphenylalaninemia. The disorders are dihydropteridine reductase (DHPR) deficiency, 6-pyruvoyltetrahydropterin synthase (6-PTS) deficiency, and guanosine triphosphate cyclohydrolase I (GTC-I) deficiency. Their initial features can resemble classic PKU or show hypotonia in the neonatal period. Progression to mental retardation, seizures, myoclonus, and motor impairment occurs even after initiation of a phenylalanine-restricted diet.

A marked increase in the urine ratio of neopterin to biopterin suggests a defect in 6-PTS, whereas a low tetrahydrobiopterin concentration is more consistent with DHPR deficiency. Administration of tetrahydrobiopterin consistently lowers blood phenylalanine concentrations. Always assay for DHPR; measure other enzymes when indicated. Therapy with tetrahydrobiopterin for the 6-PTS deficiency and with folic acid for the DHPR deficiency, together with dietary phenylalanine restriction and the administration of L-dopa, carbidopa, and 5-hydroxytryptophan are effective in some children.

Diagnosis   Newborn screening is effective in the diagnosis of PAH deficiency. Three methods of newborn screening are available. The Guthrie card bacterial inhibition assay (BIA) is inexpensive, simple, and reliable. Other tests are fluorometric analysis, which has fewer false-positive results, and tandem mass spectroscopy. An NIH Consensus Conference (2000) concluded that replacing the BIA with other tests was not cost effective.

PKU is diagnosed in individuals with plasma phenylalanine concentrations higher than 1000 μmol/L in the untreated state; non-PKU HPA is diagnosed in individuals with plasma phenylalanine concentrations consistently above normal (i.e. >120 μmol/L), but higher than 1000 μmol/L when on a normal diet. The main uses of molecular genetic testing are genetic counseling and prenatal testing.

Quantitative measurement of phenylalanine and tyrosine in the blood establishes the diagnosis. A phenylalanine concentration of greater than 20 mg/dL with a normal or reduced tyrosine concentration and urinary excretion of phenylketones is diagnostic of classic PKU. Inability to tolerate a phenylalanine challenge and normal tetrahydrobiopterin concentrations and metabolism differentiate classic PKU from the PKU variants.

Management   The treatment for PKU is to maintain the plasma phenylalanine concentrations in the near normal range (4–6 mg/dL) by dietary restriction. Initiation of dietary therapy by 3 weeks of age prevents severe, irreversible brain damage. Dietary therapy is complicated and management requires experience. The plasma phenylalanine concentration should be monitored weekly or biweekly to evaluate control (Burgard et al., 1999). The goal is to provide a complete diet that fulfills the phenylalanine requirements for normal growth and development while avoiding all significant nutrient deficiencies. Although treated patients can have normal intelligence, some have behavioral problems, learning disabilities, and attention deficit disorders. Most adults, treated early for PKU, function well. Many children with classic PKU will require life long treatment to prevent a subsequent decline in intellectual function. No established means is available to identify individuals who can safely discontinue diet therapy.

Hyperammonemia and disorders of urea synthesis

Urea synthesis is the major pathway for the metabolism of ammonia (Summar and Tuchman, 2004). The main causes of neonatal hyperammonemia are liver disease and disorders of urea synthesis. The typical initial feature of neonatal hyperammonemia is an acute overwhelming neurological disorder, exacerbated by protein feeding. Deficiency states of each enzyme responsible for catalyzing the five steps of urea synthesis exist. However, only defects in the first four steps cause clinical symptoms in the newborn: carbamyl phosphate synthetase deficiency, ornithine transcarbamylase deficiency, citrullinemia, and argininosuccinic aciduria. Arginase deficiency does not produce symptoms in the newborn. Discussion of these syndromes, as well as transitory hyperammonemia of the premature, is in this section. The hyperglycinemias are also associated with hyperammonemia but discussed in the sections that follow.

Hyperammonemia

- **Pathophysiology.** The main source of ammonia in the newborn is protein catabolism from milk. Ammonia is neurotoxic and promotes cellular swelling and brain edema. Disturbances of urea cycle metabolism are the most common cause of severe hyperammonemia in the newborn (Table 7–2).

TABLE 7–2   Neonatal hyperammonemia

Liver failure
Severe perinatal asphyxia
Total parenteral nutrition
Primary enzyme defects in urea synthesis
   Argininosuccinic acidemia
   Carbamyl phosphate synthetase deficiency
   Citrullinemia
   Ornithine transcarbamylase deficiency
Other disorders of amino acid metabolism
   Glycine encephalopathy
   Isovaleric acidemia
   Methylmalonic acidemia
   Multiple carboxylase deficiency
   Propionic acidemia
Transitory hyperammonemia of the premature infant

Other metabolic diseases can cause hyperammonemia by a secondary effect on urea metabolism. These disorders are usually associated with hypoglycemia, organic acidemia, or lactic acidosis.

- **Clinical features.** Infants with urea cycle disorders may initially appear normal, but soon after first exposure to protein feedings, ammonia accumulates and causes lethargy, hypotonia, feeding problems, vomiting, and respiratory irregularity. Coma and seizures follow. Seizures are never an initial feature, the newborn is already sick. In partial urea cycle enzyme deficiencies, illnesses or stress may trigger hyperammonemia at almost any time of life.
- **Diagnosis.** Measure the ammonia blood concentration in every newborn with a progressive encephalopathy. A plasma ammonia concentration higher than 150 mmol/L associated with a normal anion gap and a normal serum glucose concentration, indicates a urea cycle disorder. Further evaluation includes analyses of plasma amino acids, lactate, and pyruvate; and urine measurements for organic and amino acids. The combination of lactic acidosis and hyperammonemia indicates an organic acidemia or a disorder of pyruvate metabolism. Measuring the blood concentrations of citrulline, argininosuccinate, arginine, and orotic acid distinguishes specific urea cycle defects. Reduced plasma concentration of arginine may occur in all urea cycle disorders, except arginine deficiency, in which it is elevated. Molecular genetic testing is available for most deficiencies.
- **Management.** Immediate hemodialysis quickly lowers blood ammonia concentrations. Several measures dispose of waste nitrogen atoms through alternative metabolic pathways pending a specific diagnosis (Table 7–3). Initiate specific therapy within two hours of birth when prenatal diagnosis established a specific diagnosis.

TABLE 7–3   Therapy for hyperammonemia

Therapy for severe neonatal hyperammonemia of unknown cause
Peritoneal dialysis for ammonia >200 μmol/liter
No nitrogen intake until diagnosis established
10% dextrose infusion
Biotin, 10 mg/kg/day
Vitamin B$_{12}$, 1 mg/day
L-carnitine, 40 mg/kg/day IV or 100–200 mg/kg/day PO
Sodium benzoate, 0.25 g/kg initially; then 0.25–0.50 g/kg/day, constant infusion, decreasing to the lower dose if ammonia levels decrease
Arginine hydrochloride, 0.2–0.8 mg/kg initially; then 0.2–0.8 g/kg/day constant infusion with the higher dose for citrullinemia or argininosuccinic academia
Sodium phenylacetate, 0.25 g/kg initially; then 0.25–0.5 g/kg/day constant infusion decreasing to the lower dose if ammonia levels decrease

Maintenance therapy for urea cycle disorders (varies according to specific diagnosis)
Protein-restricted diet (protein, 0.75 g/kg/day)
Essential amino acids plus arginine, 0.75 g/kg/day
Sodium benzoate, 0.25–0.50 g/kg/day

Chronic therapy depends on the specific cause. Best management is by experts in the field. Therapy must balance the need for adequate protein, arginine, and energy to promote growth against the adverse effects of hyperammonemia and hyperglutaninemia. Monitoring growth and plasma concentrations of glutamine and ammonia are important for optimal therapy. In all urea cycle defects, except for arginase deficiency, arginine becomes an essential amino acid and is a dietary requirement. Liver transplantation is an alternative approach that offers a potential cure for some diseases.

Carbamyl phosphate synthetase I (CPSI) deficiency

- **Pathophysiology.** CPSI catalyzes the first step in the urea cycle; the production of carbamyl phosphate from ammonia, carbon dioxide, and adenosine triphosphate (ATP). The gene for CPS maps to chromosome locus 2q35. CPS deficiency is one of the less common defects of urea synthesis.
- **Clinical features.** The clinical presentation in the newborn is variable and depends on the completeness of enzyme deficiency. In the complete absence of CPS activity, progressive lethargy, hypotonia, and vomiting develop on the first day postpartum, even before initiating protein feedings. Loss of consciousness is progressive and generalized seizures occur on the second or third day; death follows quickly. Vomiting and lethargy correlate well with plasma ammonia concentrations greater than 200 µg/dL. Newborns with low residual levels of CPS activity have similar but less severe symptoms. Vomiting and lethargy relate closely to the time of feeding.
- **Diagnosis.** Suspect CPS deficiency in newborns with hyperammonemia and the absence of organic acidemia and aminoaciduria. Propionic acidemia, which inhibits CPS, requires specific exclusion. Plasma concentrations of glutamine are increased, but the concentration of orotic acid is normal. CPS deficiency is quickly distinguished from other defects in the urea cycle by the absence of orotic acid in the urine. The definitive diagnosis depends on enzyme assay in hepatic tissue or in leukocytes.
- **Treatment.** The duration of survival is variable. The use of a low-protein diet containing 0.6 g/kg/day of natural protein and 0.6 g/kg/day of essential amino acids prolongs survival. Administration of sodium benzoate, sodium phenylacetate, and phenylbutyrate reduces ammonia production by producing other nitrogenous products that the kidneys excrete. Even with optimal therapy, growth retardation and developmental delay in survivors are the rule.

Ornithine transcarbamylase deficiency

- **Pathophysiology.** Ornithine transcarbamylase (OTC) is the enzyme responsible for catalyzing the production of citrulline by the combination of carbamyl phosphate and ornithine. The enzyme defect is transmitted as an X-linked dominant trait (Xp21.1). Enzyme activity is completely absent in the hemizygous male and partial deficiency occurs in the heterozygous female. In one family, two consecutive males had OTC deficiency, but the mother had normal biochemical studies (Bowling et al., 1999). OTC genotyping in both brothers showed a new mutation. Genotyping of the mother showed no mutation, strongly suggesting gonadal mosaicism.

- **Clinical features.** In the hemizygous male, the clinical features resemble the syndrome associated with complete absence of CPS activity. The first few hours after birth are uneventful, but lethargy and poor feeding usually develop during the first day. Respirations become irregular. Hyperammonemia is associated with progressive obtundation, hypotonia, hypothermia, and seizures. The severity of illness in the female heterozygote depends upon the level of enzyme activity; this may vary from 19% to 97% of normal. None of the female heterozygotes have an overwhelming and fatal neonatal illness. Females with low levels of OTC activity experience recurrent episodes of hyperammonemia, seen as vomiting and obtundation, and will become mentally deficient unless treated with a low-protein diet. Females with only minimal enzyme deficiency have normal intellectual development and manifest symptoms (nausea and headache) only following a high-protein meal.
- **Diagnosis.** Definitive diagnosis relies on the direct measurement of OTC activity. The plasma concentrations of glutamine and orotic acid are increased, and the plasma concentration of citrulline is reduced. Female heterozygotes are detectable by measuring plasma ammonia and ornithine, and the urinary excretion of orotic acid following a protein load. Orotic aciduria differentiates OTC deficiency from CPS deficiency. In OTC deficiency, the rate of carbamyl phosphate synthesis is faster than its incorporation into the urea cycle. The carbamyl phosphate excess increases pyrimidine, synthesis which results in orotic aciduria.
- **Management.** Newborns with OTC activity less than 2% of normal die within the first week; activity as low as 14% is compatible with normal psychomotor development on a protein restricted diet. The treatment plan is identical to that described for CPS deficiency.

Citrullinemia

- **Pathophysiology.** Argininosuccinate synthetase (AS) is the enzyme responsible for producing argininosuccinic acid from the combination of citrulline, aspartate, and ATP. The gene locus maps to chromosome 9q34. Deficiency of AS may be partial or complete. The mode of inheritance is autosomal recessive (Thoene, 2004). Affected newborns have a complete absence of enzyme activity. Milder forms with later onset have preservation of some enzyme activity.
- **Clinical features.** Newborns appear normal at birth but then develop hyperammonemia. Progressive lethargy, feeding disturbances, and vomiting follow. Some develop signs of increased intracranial pressure. Intracranial pressure increases and is associated with spasticity and seizures. Even with prompt treatment, survivors often show severe neurological deficits.
- **Diagnosis.** Plasma ammonia concentrations reach 1000–3000 μmol/L. Diagnosis depends on the demonstration of elevated plasma and urine con-

centrations of citrulline. The concentration of citrulline is usually greater than 1000 μmol/L (normal <50 μmol/L) and plasma argininosuccinic acid is low or unmeasurable. Decreased argininosuccinate synthase (ASS) enzyme activity is demonstrable in fibroblasts. Gene sequence and linkage analysis are available.

- **Management.** The goals of management are reduction in plasma ammonia and control of increased intracranial pressure. An experimental treatment protocol that uses alternative means of waste nitrogen disposition (sodium benzoate and phenylacetate) is available. It requires FDA approval and special experience.

Argininosuccinic aciduria

- **Pathophysiology.** Argininosuccinate lyase is the enzyme responsible for catalyzing the cleavage of argininosuccinic acid to arginine and fumaric acid. The gene for the enzyme is located at 7cen-q11.2. At least two syndromes of enzyme deficiency are recognized which are possibly allelic: a malignant neonatal and a more benign infantile form. Inheritance of the neonatal form is by autosomal recessive transmission, and a partial defect is present in the heterozygous parents.

- **Clinical features.** The neonatal form causes an acute, overwhelming illness with symptoms similar to other urea cycle disorders: feeding difficulty, apathy, seizures, and hypotonia. Death usually occurs within the first 3 weeks. The infantile form is compatible with long survival, albeit with recurrent episodes of vomiting, coma, and seizures and with significant mental retardation. Anomalies of the skin and hair are sometimes associated.

- **Diagnosis.** The demonstration of argininosuccinic acid in the urine by most routine chromatographic techniques establishes the diagnosis of AL deficiency. Quantitative measurement of AL activity in the liver, erythrocytes, or fibroblasts provides further confirmation. Plasma concentrations of argininosuccinate, citrulline, and glutamine are elevated. Prenatal diagnosis is possible by assay of AL activity in amniotic fluid cells.

- **Management.** Prompt initiation of a protein-restricted diet supplemented with arginine can be life-saving (Maestri et al., 1995). The regime used is the same as that described for citrullinemia. Arginine supplementation stimulates production of citrulline and argininosuccinic acid for elimination as waste nitrogen.

Transitory hyperammonemia of the newborn (THAN)

A transitory symptomatic hyperammonemia may occur in newborns born at 34 to 36 weeks' gestation. The clinical features are respiratory distress and lethargy progressing to seizures and coma within 4 days after birth. Pupillary dilation is common.

Initial plasma ammonia concentrations are 800 to 3400 µg/dL but may peak as high as 7600 µg/dL. No deficiency of urea-cycle enzymes is demonstrable. Although the cause of hyperammonemia cannot be determined, affected newborns respond rapidly and completely to either exchange transfusion or dialysis. THAN survivors have normal neurological and developmental evaluations later on and do not experience recurrent episodes of hyperammonemia. This symptomatic hyperammonemia may be an exaggeration of a physiological, nonsymptomatic hyperammonemia detected in more than 50% of prematures that does not require treatment.

Glycine Encephalopathy

Many inborn errors of amino acid metabolism are associated with elevated plasma concentrations of glycine. The presence or absence of associated keto-acidosis divides the hyperglycinemias into two groups. Nonketotic hyperglycinemia (glycine encephalopathy) is a relatively homogeneous entity secondary to a defect in the glycine cleaving system. Inheritance is autosomal recessive (Applegarth et al., 2003). Ketotic hyperglycinemia is a heterogeneous entity that includes several inborn errors in the metabolism of branched-chain amino acids and their metabolites.

Glycine is a nonessential two-carbon amino acid whose major metabolic pathways are involved in the synthesis of other molecules. Several of these pathways require the interconversion of glycine and serine. The glycine cleavage system accomplishes the interconversion. This system, confined to the mitochondria, is composed of four protein components. Chromosome 9p22 encodes the P-protein, a pyridoxal phosphate-dependent glycine decarboxylase. Defects in the P protein cause nonketotic hyperglycinemia 1 (NKH1). The T-protein is a tetrahydrofolate-requiring enzyme encoded on chromosome 3p21.2-p21.1 (NKH2). The H-protein contains lipoic acid (NKH3) and the L-protein is lipoamide dehydrogenase. Defects of one or more of these proteins causes elevated glycine concentrations in the blood, urine, cerebrospinal fluid, and brain. NKH 1 and 2 account for most clinical cases. Transmission of all is by autosomal recessive inheritance.

- **Clinical features.** Affected newborns are normal at birth but become irritable and refuse feeding anytime from 6 hours to 8 days after delivery. The onset of symptoms is usually within 48 hours but delays by a few weeks occur in milder allelic forms. Hiccupping is an early and continuous feature; some mothers relate that the child hiccupped in utero. Progressive lethargy, hypotonia, respiratory disturbances, and myoclonic seizures follow. Some newborns survive the acute illness, but mental retardation, epilepsy, and spasticity characterize the subsequent course.

  In the milder forms range, the onset of seizures is after the neonatal period. The developmental outcome is better, but does not exceed moderate mental retardation.
- **Diagnosis.** During the acute encephalopathy, the EEG demonstrates a burst-suppression pattern, which evolves during infancy into hypsarrhythmia.

MRI shows partial agenesis of the corpus callosum. Hyperglycinemia and especially elevated concentrations of glycine in the cerebrospinal fluid, in the absence of hyperammonemia or organic acidemia, establishes the diagnosis.

- **Management.** No therapy has proven to be effective. Hemodialysis provides only temporary relief of the encephalopathy, and diet therapy has not proved successful in modifying the course. Diazepam, a competitor for glycine receptors, in combination with choline, folic acid, and sodium benzoate, may stop the seizures. Oral administration of sodium benzoate at doses of 250–750 mg/kg/day can reduce the plasma glycine concentration into the normal range. This substantially reduces but does not normalize CSF glycine concentration. Carnitine, 100 mg/kg/day, may increase the glycine conjugation with benzoate.

Disorders of Branched-chain Amino Acids and Ketoacids

The three major branched-chain amino acids are leucine, isoleucine, and valine. Propionyl-CoA and methylmalonyl-CoA are products of their metabolism (Fig. 7–1). Several inborn errors in the metabolism of branched-chain amino acids and ketoacids are recognized; most produce disorders in the newborn.

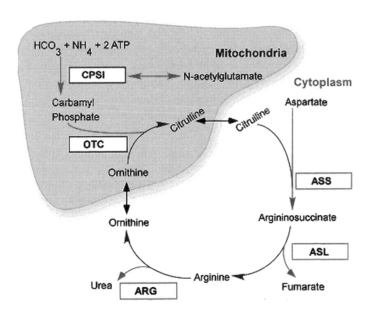

FIGURE 7–1. Urea cycle disorders. Urea cycle disorders overview. In: GeneClinics: Medical Genetics Knowledge Base. [database online]. University of Washington, Seattle. Available at http://www.geneclinics.org. From Summar ML, Tuchman M. (Updated 21 June 2004).

Maple Syrup Urine Disease (MSUD)

- **Pathophysiology.** An almost complete absence (less than 2% of normal) of branched-chain ketoacid dehydrogenase (BCKD) causes the neonatal form of maple syrup urine disease (MSUD). BCKD is composed of six subunits, but the main abnormality in MSUD is deficiency of the E1 subunit on chromosome 19q13.1-q13.2. Leucine, isoleucine, and valine cannot be decarboxylated, and accumulate in blood, urine, and tissues (Fig. 7–1).
- **Clinical features.** MSUD presents as an acute overwhelming illness. Affected newborns appear healthy at birth but develop feeding difficulties and a shrill cry during the first week. The Moro reflex is absent and tone alternates between flaccidity and spasticity. Signs of increased intracranial pressure, split sutures, and bulging fontanelle may be present due to cerebral edema. Hyperleucinemia induces hypoglycemia. Opisthotonos, seizures, and coma follow. Death usually occurs by the end of the first month, although some infants survive beyond 1 year. A maple syrup odor in the urine is detectable on the fifth day and is usually pervasive in all body secretions by the second week. A polymer of alpha-hydroxybutyric acid (a constituent of natural maple syrup) derived from alpha-ketobutyric acid causes the odor.
- **Diagnosis.** Plasma amino acid concentrations show increased plasma concentrations of the three branch-chained amino acids. Measures of enzyme in lymphocytes or cultured fibroblasts serve as a confirmatory test. Heterozygotes are detectable by diminished levels of enzyme activity in cultured fibroblasts and by their response to an oral leucine tolerance test. In MSUD homozygotes, a leucine load of 150 mg/kg produces prolonged hyperleucinemia and profound hypoglycemia. The same leucine load in heterozygotes also causes leucinemia, which is less severe but is still distinctly abnormal.
- **Management.** Exchange transfusions or peritoneal dialysis in critically ill newborns transiently lower the plasma concentration of branched-chain amino acids and ketoacids, but the additional administration of insulin and glucose provides a more prolonged reduction, presumably by promoting the uptake of amino acids into skeletal muscle. Discontinue the intake of all natural protein immediately and correct dehydration, electrolyte imbalance, and metabolic acidosis. The provision of intravenous glucose, lipids, and BCAA-free amino acids promotes an anabolic state. A trial of thiamine, 10–20 mg/kg per day, documents a thiamine-responsive MSUD variant.

A diet low in leucine, isoleucine, and valine with amino acids added to the base mix to provide 75 to 100 mg/kg/day each of leucine, isoleucine, and valine is experimental. The maximum daily tolerance for valine is approximately 140 mg/kg. Leucine blood levels are very labile and require close monitoring. The overall success of diet therapy is variable and inversely related to the age of treatment initiation.

There is a tendency among physicians to withhold all feedings from children who are acutely ill and vomiting and to manage acidosis with fluids and electrolytes alone. However, newborns and infants with MSUD may do better during acute attacks if given a nasal gastric drip of their prepared diet, rather than with intravenous therapy alone.

Isovaleric Acidemia

- **Pathophysiology.** Isovaleric acid is a fatty acid derived from leucine. Its conversion to propionyl-CoA is metabolized by the enzyme isovaleryl-CoA dehydrogenase. The enzyme is encoded on chromosome 15q14-q15 Deficiency of the dehydrogenase is transmitted by autosomal recessive inheritance, and the heterozygous state can be detected in cultured fibroblasts.
- **Clinical features.** Newborns are normal at birth but within a few days, become lethargic, refuse to feed, and vomit. The clinical syndrome is very similar to MSUD. A major difference between the two is body odor. In isovaleric acidemia, the odor is described as that of 'sweaty feet' rather than that of maple syrup. Most will die within 3 weeks of ketoacidosis, hemorrhagic diatheses due to pancytopenia, or an intercurrent infection. The hemorrhagic diathesis may lead to intracranial hemorrhage.
- **Diagnosis.** Serum concentrations of lactate and isovaleric acids are elevated, as are urine concentrations of isovaleric acid and isovaleryl glycine. Isovaleryl-CoA dehydrogenase activity can be assayed in cultured skin fibroblasts.
- **Management.** Management is similar to that described for MSUD, Protein restriction and carnitine administration are the main intervention. Acylcarnitine is formed and excreted in the urine to eliminate toxic metabolites. Carnitine also increases protein tolerance and provides some protection from encephalopathy during acute illnesses. Glucose infusion during acute attacks reduces protein catabolism. Although glycine is recommended, carnitine supplementation alone is satisfactory in some patients.

Multiple Carboxylase Deficiency

- **Pathophysiology.** Holocarboxylase synthetase covalently links biotin to propionyl-CoA-carboxylase, pyruvate carboxylase, and 3-methylcrotonyl-CoA carboxylase. The enzyme is encoded on chromosome 21q22.1. In the neonatal form of multiple carboxylase deficiency (MCD), deficiency of holocarboxylase synthetase causes an organic acidemia.
- **Clinical features.** Lethargy, vomiting, and hypotonia are the typical features. Coma and death follow if treatment is not initiated promptly.
- **Diagnosis.** The diagnosis is confirmed by holocarboxylase synthetase enzyme activities in leukocytes.
- **Management.** Holocarboxylase deficiency responds to biotin, 10 mg per day.

Propionic Acidemia

- **Pathophysiology.** Propionyl-CoA carboxylase, the enzyme responsible for catalyzing the formation of D-methylmalonyl-CoA, requires the coenzyme biotin. Propionic acidemia is due to deficient activity of the enzyme propionyl-CoA carboxylase. Because propionyl-CoA requires biotin as a cofactor, disorders of biotin also cause propionic acidemia.
- **Clinical features.** Most affected children appear normal at birth; symptoms may begin as early as the first day postpartum but can be delayed for months or years. In the newborn, the symptoms are nonspecific: feeding difficulty, lethargy, hypotonia, and dehydration. The subsequent course is characterized by recurrent attacks of profound metabolic acidosis, often associated with hyperammonemia, which respond poorly to buffering. Untreated newborns rapidly become dehydrated, have generalized or myoclonic seizures, and become comatose. Hepatomegaly due to fatty infiltration occurs in some patients. Neutropenia, thrombocytopenia, and occasionally pancytopenia may be present as well. A bleeding diathesis accounts for massive intracranial hemorrhage in some newborns.
- **Diagnosis.** Propionic acidemia should be considered in any newborn with ketoacidosis but must also be considered in newborns with hyperammonemia and without ketoacidosis, an erroneous diagnosis of carbamyl phosphate synthesis deficiency may be suggested. Measuring blood and urine concentrations of organic and amino acids shows a characteristic biochemical profile. Typical findings include high concentrations of propionic acid, 3-hydroxypropionate, methylcitrate, 3-hydroxyvaleric acid, and propionylglycine. Measuring the enzyme activity in fibroblasts makes the definitive diagnosis. Prenatal diagnosis can be accomplished by the detection of methylcitrate, a unique metabolite or propionate, in the amniotic fluid, and by demonstration of deficient enzyme activity in amniotic fluid cells.
- **Management.** The newborn in metabolic crisis may require peritoneal or hemodialysis to remove toxic metabolites. Large amounts of parenteral fluids are required to prevent dehydration. An adequate caloric intake must be provided by glucose, as all protein must be eliminated during the acute attack. The frequency and severity of subsequent attacks are decreased, but not completely abolished, by restricting protein intake to 1 to 1.2 g/kg/day. Oral administration of L-carnitine reduces the ketogenic response to fasting and may be useful as a daily supplement. Biotin supplementation has been used in several patients without any clear indication that it favorably influences the course of the disease. However, there may be a subset of patients that are responsive.

Methylmalonic Acidemia

- **Pathophysiology.** D-methylmalonyl-CoA is racemized to L-methylmalonyl-CoA by the enzyme D-methylmalonyl racemase and then isomerized to succinyl-CoA, which enters the TCA cycle. The enzyme D-methylmalonyl-CoA mutase catalyzes isomerization, with the cobalamin (vitamin B_{12})

coenzyme adenosylcobalamin required as a cofactor. Seven biochemical forms of methylmalonic acidemia have been identified. The net effect of each is to block the conversion of methylmalonyl-CoA to succinyl-CoA. Propionyl-CoA, propionic acid, and methylmalonic acid accumulate and cause hyperglycinemia and hyperammonemia. Each of the enzyme defects is transmitted as an autosomal recessive trait.

- **Clinical features.** The typical onset in the newborn is a catastrophic encephalopathy after introducing protein feedings. Children with complete mutase deficiency have the poorest prognosis and frequently die during an acute episode.
- **Diagnosis.** The biochemical features include severe ketoacidosis, hypoglycemia, hyperammonemia, lactic acidosis, and secondary carnitine deficiency. The blood and urine glycine concentrations are increased. Urine organic acid analysis shows high concentrations of methylmalonic acid and lower concentrations of 3-hydroxypropionate, methylcitrate, and other metabolites of propionyl-CoA. Definitive diagnosis requires enzyme analysis of cultured fibroblasts or gene identification.
- **Management.** Intramuscular hydroxocobalamin (1.0–2.0 mg/day) can reverse many of the clinical and biochemical features (Andersson and Shapira, 1998). L-Carnitine supplementation is indicated for both acute and chronic management.

DISORDERS OF CARBOHYDRATE METABOLISM

Among this relatively rare group of disorders, the most common manifestation of neurological dysfunction in the newborn is seizures secondary to hypoglycemia. These seizures frequently occur against a background of systemic illness and are usually related to the time of feeding.

Fructosemia

- **Pathophysiology.** Fructose is widely distributed in fruits and vegetables either as the free monosaccharide or as part of the disaccharide sucrose. It is rapidly cleared from the blood, phosphorylated in the liver, and then converted to pyruvate and its metabolites. The two main disorders of fructose metabolism are *hereditary fructose intolerance* (HFI), caused by deficiency of the enzyme is aldolase B, and *fructose bisphosphatase deficiency* (FBD). Both are transmitted by autosomal recessive inheritance and rarely cause symptoms in the newborn, because newborns are not ordinarily exposed to fructose.

  HFI catalyzes the cleavage of fructose-1-phosphate to form dihydroxyacetone phosphate and D-glyceraldehyde. Absence of the enzyme results in the accumulation of fructose 1-phosphate. Increased concentrations of fructose-1-phosphate inhibit fructokinase, the enzyme responsible for the phosphorylation of fructose, and thereby cause fructosemia and fructosuria.

Fructosemia depresses the blood level of glucose. Fructose does not penetrate the blood–brain barrier and cannot substitute for glucose as a substrate for cerebral metabolism. FBD impairs gluconeogenesis in a similar manner (Kikawa et al., 1995).

- **Clinical features.** The onset of symptoms is typically related to the first ingestion of fructose, usually in the form of a fruit juice supplement to feeding. Hypoglycemia is almost immediate; the child vomits and becomes lethargic, the state of consciousness declines, and seizures follow (Edstrom, 1990). Continued ingestion of fructose causes failure to thrive and repeated episodes of hypoglycemia, vomiting, hepatomegaly, jaundice, ascites, hyperbilirubinemia, albuminuria, and aminoaciduria. The severity of symptoms depends upon the amount of fructose ingested and the degree of enzyme deficiency.
- **Diagnosis.** Urine test results for reducing substances are positive; however, the glucose oxidase test result is negative. Qualitative chromatography is necessary to identify urine fructose. The hepatic enzymes fructose bisphosphate aldolase and fructose bisphosphatase can be measured for a specific diagnosis.
- **Management.** All the clinical features are rapidly reversed by the removal of sucrose and fructose from the diet. Untreated infants develop hepatic dysfunction and brain damage.

Galactosemia

Three separate inborn errors of galactose metabolism are known to produce galactosemia in the newborn: galactose-1-phosphate uridyltransferase (GALT) deficiency, galactokinase (kinase) deficiency, and uridine diphosphate galactose-4-epimerase (epimerase) deficiency. All three defects are transmitted by autosomal recessive inheritance. GALT deficiency is the most common inborn error of metabolism associated with galactosemia, and is the only disturbance of galactose metabolism that produces neurological symptoms in the newborn. Kinase deficiency causes the development of cataracts during infancy and childhood, and epimerase deficiency is asymptomatic. Disturbances in kinase and epimerase, although infrequent, can be detected in newborn screening tests for galactosemia and need to be differentiated from GALT deficiency.

- **Pathophysiology.** The principal carbohydrate of mammalian milk is the disaccharide lactose. Lactose is hydrolyzed in the intestine to its component hexoses: glucose and galactose. Galactose is phosphorylated to galactose-1-phosphate and is then converted to glucose-1-phosphate. This conversion is blocked in GALT deficiency. GALT catalyzes the production of glucose-1-phosphate and uridyldiphosphate (UDP)-galactose from galactose-1-phosphate and UPD-glucose.

   GALT is present in most mammalian tissues. It is inhibited by glucose-1-phosphate and may also be influenced, to some degree, by the concentration of other carbohydrate metabolites. In the GALT deficiency state, galactose-1-phosphate, galactose, and galactitol accumulate in the blood and tissues. Galactitol is a reduction product formed from excess galactose through an alternate metabolic pathway.

- **Diagnosis.** Galactosemia can be detected in all affected newborns by screening programs. The definitive diagnosis is established by measurement of erythrocyte GALT activity and by isoelectric focusing of GALT (Elsas, 1999). Affected individuals have GALT activity that is less than 5% of control values. A less severe form is called the *Duarte variant* in which GALT activity is 5 to 20% of control values. Molecular genetic testing of the GALT gene (chromosomal locus 9p13) is available for prognostication, heterozygote detection, genetic counseling, and prenatal diagnosis. In the absence of screening, galactosemia should be considered in any newborn with vomiting and hepatomegaly and should be strongly suspected when cataracts are associated.
- **Clinical features.** Affected newborns appear healthy at birth, but have already begun to form nuclear cataracts. Both galactose-1-phosphate and galactitol are found in the lens. Galactitol is probably the critical compound in the pathogenesis of cataracts. Newborns with kinase deficiency develop cataracts in the absence of galactose-1-phosphate. The initial features of GALT deficiency (poor suck, failure to thrive, vomiting, and diarrhea) begin shortly after the first milk feeding. By the end of the first week, jaundice and hepatomegaly are present as well. Ascites, splenomegaly, bleeding diathesis, and jaundice are associated. Hyperammonemia, sepsis, and shock follow (Waggoner et al., 1990). Increased intracranial pressure, evidenced by a bulging anterior fontanelle, is the most common feature of neurological dysfunction. Mental retardation is a constant outcome in untreated children.
- **Management.** Early dietary treatment prevents most complications. All symptoms are reversible, even after many months, by the removal of lactose from the diet. Vomiting and diarrhea cease, appetite increases, liver function improves, and cataract formation reverses. Constructing a lactose-free diet is difficult because lactose is abundant in most foods. However, soybean formulas are considered safe to use throughout infancy, and satisfactory diets have been designed for childhood. Dietary restrictions on all lactose-containing foods should continue throughout life. Calcium supplements of 500 mg/day are recommended in the neonatal period and >1200 mg/day in childhood (Elsas and Acosta, 1998). With early diagnosis and dietary therapy, normal physical and intellectual growth is possible; with each month that diagnosis is delayed, the probability of mental retardation is increased.

Disorders of Glycogen Metabolism

Glycogen is the principal form of carbohydrate storage in animals and is found, to some degree, in all tissues of the body. Cerebral storage of glycogen is minimal. The brain relies on a constant supply of blood glucose for energy, rather than on carbohydrate stores. Therefore, when there is a disorder of glycogen metabolism, cerebral dysfunction more commonly results from hypoglycemia than from abnormal neuronal storage. However, weakness and hypotonia may be prominent in glycogen storage diseases affecting muscle. Disorders of glycogen metabolism usually present as primary disturbances of the liver, heart, or musculoskeletal system. Only two disorders cause symptoms in the newborn: glucose-6-phosphatase deficiency and acid maltase deficiency.

Glucose-6-phosphatase Deficiency (Von Gierke's Disease)

- **Pathophysiology.** Glucose-6-phosphate, a major intermediary of glucose metabolism, can be converted either to glucose or to pyruvate. Glucose-6-phosphatase is a microsomal enzyme responsible for catalyzing the conversion of glucose-6-phosphate to glucose. As all glucose derived from gluconeogenesis must come from glucose-6-phosphate, deficiency of the enzyme precludes glucose production from any endogenous source. Thus, relatively short periods of fasting result in hypoglycemia. A further consequence of this metabolic block is the diversion of glucose-6-phosphate to pyruvate and then to lactic acid. Tertiary events include hyperglucagonemia, hyperalaninemia, hyperglyceridemia, and hyperuricemia. Glucose-6-phosphatase deficiency is transmitted by autosomal recessive inheritance.
- **Clinical features.** Hepatomegaly is the only common manifestation of glucose-6-phosphatase deficiency in the newborn. Hypoglycemic seizures sometimes occur in the first month postpartum but more often have their onset during infancy. The liver feels smooth and firm to palpation and may extend down to the iliac crest. Splenomegaly and cardiomegaly are not present. Bleeding time is prolonged because of abnormal platelet aggregation. Growth and development are frequently retarded.
- **Management.** Total parenteral nutrition, nocturnal nasogastric infusions of glucose, or frequent oral administration of uncooked cornstarch have been used to maintain blood glucose concentrations. The use of uncooked cornstarch achieves satisfactory glucose concentrations for 2.5 to 6 hours (Lee et al., 1996). Continuous nocturnal intragastric infusion combined with frequent feedings during daytime is now the therapy of choice in glucose-6-phosphatase deficiency and has been demonstrated to reverse both the clinical symptoms and the biochemical abnormalities.

Acid Maltase Deficiency (Pompe's Disease)

- **Pathophysiology.** Pompe's disease is transmitted by autosomal recessive inheritance. The abnormal gene is located on chromosome 17. Acid maltase is a lysosomal enzyme, present in all tissues, that hydrolyzes maltose and catalyzes the transglucosylation from maltose to glycogen. It is not required for glycolysis and is not a factor in the maintenance of normal blood glucose concentrations. The deficiency state results in a massive accumulation of glycogen within lysosomes, leading to cell damage and necrosis. Infants with Pompe's disease store glycogen in several tissues, especially muscle, heart, and lower motor neurons. Affected tissues have cytoplasmic vacuoles containing material that stains with the periodic acid–Schiff reagent. The vacuoles are membrane-bound and can be identified as distended lysosomes.

- **Clinical features.** Three distinct clinical forms are associated with acid maltase deficiency: infantile, childhood, and adult. The infantile form is the most severe, causing glycogen storage in all tissues. In the childhood and adult forms, skeletal muscle is the major target organ. The initial features of the infantile form, profound hypotonia and cardiomegaly, may be present in the newborn, but more usually appear during the second month. The electrocardiogram (EKG) shows short PR intervals and high QRS complexes on all leads. Death from cardiac failure usually occurs by 6 months of age.
- **Diagnosis.** Acid maltase deficiency should be considered in hypotonic infants with cardiomegaly or heart failure. Muscle biopsy specimens show characteristic large vacuoles containing material that stains positive on periodic acid–Schiff. Definitive diagnosis requires measuring the enzyme concentration in muscle, leukocytes, or cultured fibroblasts.
- **Treatment.** Treatment is not available.

Disorders of Oxidative Metabolism and Mitochondria

Mitochondria are subcellular organelles that support oxidative metabolism. Most structural components of the mitochondria are encoded on nuclear DNA, but 3% of mitochondrial proteins are encoded by maternally inherited mitochondrial DNA (mtDNA). mtDNA encodes 13 proteins in the respiratory chain. The brain, retina, peripheral nerves, heart, and skeletal muscles are the ones most dependent on mitochondrial energy production and are the ones most often affected in mitochondrial disease. Disturbances of mitochondrial DNA cause multisystem disorders with variable phenotypes among members of the same family. Lactic acidosis is the most common feature of mitochondrial disorders in the newborn.

Pyruvate is at the very center of intermediary metabolism. It is formed primarily from glucose by the process of glycolysis and is used by one of four processes: (1) transamination to alanine; (2) reduction to lactate; (3) carboxylation to oxaloacetate, an intermediary in the tricarboxylic acid (TCA) cycle, catalyzed by the enzyme pyruvate carboxylase; and (4) oxidative decarboxylation to CO_2 and acetyl-coenzyme A, catalyzed by the pyruvate dehydrogenase enzyme complex (PDH).

Lactic Acidosis

- **Pathophysiology.** Lactic acid is the normal end product of anaerobic glucose metabolism. Lactic acidosis occurs during anoxia-ischemia and in metabolic failure from liver disease or diabetes mellitus. Inborn errors of metabolism that cause lactic acidosis may result from oxidative metabolic defects (primary) or defects in other metabolic pathways (secondary) that impair mitochondrial metabolism. Lactic acid is the end product of pyruvate metabolism and acts as a reservoir for excess pyruvate. Lactic dehydrogenase converts lactate back to pyruvate, which is then further metabolized through the citric acid cycle. The blood lactate to pyruvate ratio is useful in the diagnosis of primary lactic acidosis. Defects of enzymes close to pyruvate in the metabolic pathway usually produce ratios of less than 20, whereas electron transport chain defects that cause NADH accumulation have ratios greater than 20.

- **Clinical features.** The main feature of primary lactic acidosis in the newborn is a metabolic encephalopathy associated with tachypnea and irritability. The encephalopathy progresses to coma, seizures, and death.
- **Diagnosis.** Blood lactate and pyruvate concentrations are measured. Reliable measurements require a free-flowing venous sample collected from indwelling catheter. Cerebrospinal fluid lactate and pyruvate concentrations may be elevated in patients with lactic acidosis even when blood levels are normal. Lactic acidosis caused by organic acid disorders or amino acid disorders must be excluded by measuring quantitative urine organic acids and blood amino acids. Blood biotinidase and ammonia also should be measured.
- **Management.** Intravenous sodium bicarbonate is needed to reverse acute, life-threatening lactic. Peritoneal dialysis with bicarbonate may be needed as well. Thiamine, riboflavin, biotin, ascorbic acid, carnitine, and coenzyme Q_{10} are often recommended.

Pyruvate Dehydrogenase Deficiency

- **Pathophysiology.** Pyruvate dehydrogenase (PDH) deficiency is a mitochondrial enzyme complex composed of five subunits. The three main components of the complex are termed E1, E2, and E3. Thiamine is a cofactor for E1 and lipoic acid for E3. A phosphatase and a kinase, respectively, activate and inactivate the E1 component. The drug dichloroacetic acid activates PDH by inhibiting the kinase. PDH is the major regulating step for entry of carbohydrate carbon skeletons into the citric acid cycle and provides the fine control needed for oxidative metabolism.
- **Clinical features.** E1 deficiency accounts for 90% of PDH deficiency. Disease severity correlates with enzyme activity. Newborns with severe deficiency show severe lactic acidosis and usually die. Those who survive are mentally retarded and may show agenesis of the corpus callosum and cystic lesions of the basal ganglia, cerebellum, and brainstem.
- **Diagnosis.** PDH deficiency should be suspected in newborns with lactic acidosis. Pyruvic acid concentrations are elevated above and the lactate to pyruvate ratio is low. Definitive diagnosis requires enzymatic study of muscle, leukocytes, or fibroblasts.
- **Management.** Thiamine is given because it is a cofactor for E1. The use of dichloroacetate is under study. Lactic acidosis is treated as described in the previous section.

Pyruvate Carboxylase and Biotinidase Deficiency

- **Pathophysiology.** Pyruvate carboxylase (PC) catalyzes the condensation of CO_2 with pyruvate to form oxaloacetate and thereby supplies 4-carbon skeletons to the citric acid cycle. Biotin is an essential cofactor and deficiency of biotin or of biotinidase reduces PC activity.

- **Clinical features.** Absence of PC causes severe neonatal lactic acidosis, hypoglycemia, and elevated blood alanine, citrulline, lysine, and ammonia concentrations. 2-Oxoglutaric acid is increased in the urine. Lipid accumulation causes hepatomegaly. Death occurs by 3 months of age.
- **Diagnosis.** PC deficiency should be considered in children with lactic acidosis and hypoglycemia. Definitive diagnosis requires PC measurement in leukocytes or fibroblasts.
- **Management.** Biotin supplementation, 10–20 mg per day, is recommended.

DISORDERS OF LIPID METABOLISM

Disturbances in the metabolism of lipids are a major cause of progressive neurological deterioration in infancy. However, the onset of clinical manifestations rarely occurs before 3 months of age, even though the pathological process is advanced in the fetus. Only two disorders of lipid metabolism have clinical manifestations at birth or during the first month: infantile G_{M1} gangliosidosis and the acute neuronopathic form of Gaucher's disease. The neonatal forms of both diseases have multisystem involvement.

Infantile G_{M1} Gangliosidosis Type I

- **Pathophysiology.** Abnormal storage of G_{M1} gangliosides may present at birth (infantile type I) or during infancy (juvenile type II). Both diseases are hereditary deficiencies of the enzyme acid-β-galactosidase encoded by on chromosome 3p21.33 and are transmitted as autosomal-recessive traits. In type I, all three isoenzymes of β-galactosidase are missing while in type II; only the B and C isoenzymes are deficient. G_{M1} accumulates in the brain and viscera; a galactose-containing glycoprotein that resembles keratin sulfate accumulates in the viscera as well.
- **Clinical features.** Edema of face and limbs, hepatosplenomegaly, failure to thrive, and retarded psychomotor development are present from birth. Appetite is poor, and the sucking reflex is weak; hypotonia is generalized. The face has a characteristic appearance typified by frontal bossing, depressed nasal bridge, large low-set ears, increased nasolabial distance, gingival hypertrophy, macroglossia, and hirsutism. A cherry-red spot, identical to that observed in Tay–Sachs disease, is observed in the macular region. The cornea is normal. Recurrent seizures and progressive neurological deterioration characterize the subsequent course. Few infants survive the second year.
- **Management.** Therapy is supportive.

Gaucher's Disease

- **Pathophysiology.** Gaucher's disease is the most common sphingolipido-sis. It results from deficient activity of glucocerebrosidase (gene map locus 1q21), the enzyme responsible for catalyzing the cleavage of glucose from glucocerebroside. Three clinical forms have been recognized and identified as types I, II, and III. Type II, the acute neuronopathic form, is the only one that can have clinical manifestations at birth.
- **Clinical features.** The clinical triad of Gaucher's disease is hepatospleno-megaly, progressive neurological deterioration, and hyperextension of the neck. Difficulty in feeding or swallowing and failure to thrive are early symptoms. Persistent retroflexion of the head is a common but unexplained finding. Other neurological signs are strabismus, spasticity, hyperactive deep tendon reflexes, and seizures. The progress of the disease is most rapid when symptoms begin at birth. Death usually occurs within 6 months from respira-tory complications, but patients may survive up to 2 years of age.
- **Management.** Intravenous enzyme replacement therapy is effective in type I disease but not in type II.

REFERENCES AND FURTHER READING

Applegarth DA, Toone J and Hamosh A. Glycine encephalopathy. (16 May 2003) In: GeneClinics: Medical Genetics Knowledge Base. [database online] University of Washington, Seattle. Available at http://www.geneclinics.org

Andersson HC and Shapira E. Biochemical and clinical response to hydroxycobalamin versus cyanoco-balamin treatment in patients with methylmalonic acidemia and homocystinuria (cblC). J Pediatr 1998;132:121–124.

Batshaw ML. Inborn errors of urea synthesis. Ann Neurol 1994;35:133–141.

Bowling F, McGown I, McGill J, et al. Maternal gonadal mosaicism causing ornithine transcarbamylase deficiency. Am J Med Genet 1999;85:452–454.

Burgard P, Bremer HJ, Buhrdel P, et al. Rationale for the German recommendations for phenylalanine level control in phenylketonuria 1997. Eur J Pediatr 1999;158:46–54.

Elsas L and Acosta P. Nutritional support of inherited metabolic disease. In: Shils M, Olson J, Shike M and Ross AC (eds). Modern Nutrition in Health and Disease, 9th edn. Baltimore: Williams and Wilkins, 1998; pp. 1003–1056.

Edstrom CS. Hereditary fructose intolerance in the vomiting infant. Pediatrics 1990;85:600–603.

Elsas LJ II. (Updated 30 November 1999) Galactosemia. In: GeneClinics: Medical Genetics Knowledge Base. [database online]. University of Washington, Seattle. Available at http://www.geneclinics.org/profiles/galactosemia/ Accessed July 2000.

Hamosh A, Maher JF, Bellus GA, et al. Long term use of high-dose benzoate and dextromethorphan for the treatment of nonketotic hyperglycinemia. J Pediatr 1998;132:709–713.

Kikawa Y, Iuzuka M, Jin BY, et al. Identification of a genetic mutation in a family with fructose-1, 6-biphosphatase deficiency. Biochem Biophys Res Commun 1995;210:797–804.

Lee PJ, Dixon MA and Leonard JV. Uncooked cornstarch–efficacy in type I glycogenosis. Arch Dis Child 1996;74:546–547.

Maestri NE, Clissold DB and Brusilow SW. Long-term survival of patients with argininosuccinate syn-thetase deficiency. Pediatrics 1995;127:929–935.

National Institutes of Health Consensus Development Conference Statement: Phenylketonuria: screening and management, October 16–18 2000. Pediatrics 2000;108:972–982.

Ryan BS and Scriver CR. (Updated 8 July 2004). Phenylalanine hydroxylase deficiency. In: GeneClinics: Medical Genetics Knowledge Base. [database online]. University of Washington, Seattle. Available at http://www.geneclinics.org

Scriver CR. Why mutation analysis does not always predict clinical consequences: explanations in the era of genomics. J Pediatr 2002;140:502–506.

Summar ML and Tuchman M. (Updated 21 June 2004). Urea cycle disorders overview. In GeneClinics: Medical Genetics Knowledge Base. [database online]. University of Washington, Seattle. Available at http://www.geneclinics.org

Thoene JG. (Updated 7 July 2004). Citrullinemia Type 1. In: GeneClinics: Medical Genetics Knowledge Base. [database online]. University of Washington, Seattle. Available at http://www.geneclinics.org

Van Hove JLK, Kishnani P, Muenzer J, et al. Benzoate therapy and carnitine deficiency in non-ketotic hyperglycemia. Am J Med Genet 1995;59:444–453.

Waggoner DD, Buist NR and Donnell GN. Long-term prognosis in galactosaemia: Results of a survey of 350 cases. J Inherit Metab Dis 1990;13:802–818.

8

Disorders of Cerebral Morphogenesis

Gerald M. Fenichel

Previous chapters examined the neuropathology of several intrauterine disorders. Many such disorders cause destructive changes in the developing brain that result in organ malformation. The observed patterns of tissue necrosis and response do not differ significantly from their postnatal counterparts and are recognizable as the consequence of specific etiological agents. In addition, structural malformations may also arise secondary to several inborn errors of metabolism.

The malformations described in this chapter lack recognizable patterns of disease and represent primary failures of morphogenesis. Many are disturbances in the delicate sequencing of brain development caused by genetic mutations. Similar disturbances are reproducible experimentally in animals by a variety of toxic and infectious agents. Morphogenetic errors, although lacking in the traditional stigmata of tissue injury, could result from exposure of an embryo to infectious or toxic agents during the first weeks after conception. At this early stage, a noxious environmental agent could disorganize the delicate sequencing of neural development at a time when the brain is incapable of generating a cellular response. The etiology of many malformations remains uncertain, and may be multifactorial. This chapter classifies malformations by the three phases of cerebral organogenesis: (1) neurolation, the formation and closure of the neural tube, 3–4 weeks' gestation; (2) prosencephalization, the development of the forebrain 2–3 months of gestation; and (3) histogenesis, the proliferation and migration of neurons, beginning at 3 months gestation and continuing postnatally. Chapter 9 discusses primary malformations of the ventricular system, in which hydrocephalus is a prominent feature.

NEUROLATION

Neural Tube Development

At the end of the first week, a rostrocaudal axis, *the primitive streak*, is identifiable on the dorsal aspect of the embryo. A second rostrocaudal axis, *the notochord*, develops adjacent to the primitive streak. The notochord is responsible for the subsequent induction both of a dorsal neural plate and of a ventral neuroenteric canal. The primitive spinal cord and gut are therefore contiguous; this contiguity is important in understanding persistent connections from ventral defects in neurolation.

Conversion of the primitive neural plate into a closed neural tube occurs during the third and fourth weeks of gestation. Incomplete or defective formation of the neural tube, *neural tube defects*, is a common malformation of the human central nervous system with a prevalence of 0.5 to 2 per 1000 livebirths. The initial step in this conversion is the formation of the neural folds by a proliferation of cells at the lateral margin of the neural plate. The lateral proliferation creates a central indentation, *the neural groove*. The cells of the neural plate are in contact with amniotic fluid (the extra-embryonic world). A maturational arrest at this stage results in the absence of a dermal or boney covering for the central nervous system. The cells at the apex of the neural fold comprise the neural crest. These will give rise to sensory ganglia, autonomic ganglia, Schwann cells, melanocytes, and pia arachnoid. The first meeting and fusion of the neural folds to form a neural canal is at the level of the future medulla. The most rostral portion of the canal, the anterior neuropore, closes at about 24 days and then undergoes marked differentiation and cleavage (prosencephalization) to form the forebrain. The caudal progression of canalization ends with closure of the posterior neuropore (the future lumbosacral spine) at about 27 days. The mesoderm surrounding the neural tube gives rise to the dura, skull, and vertebrae, but not to the skin, which is ectodermal in origin. Therefore, defects in the final closure of the neural tube and its mesodermal case do not preclude the presence of a dermal covering.

Neural Tube Defects (1–4 Weeks' Gestation)

Midline disturbances in closure of the neural tube and its coverings are termed *dysraphia*. The most frequent location of dysraphic defects is at the extreme ends of the neural tube, the anterior and posterior neuropores, but defects may also occur at any site in between. Defective closure of the anterior neuropore results in *anencephaly*; defective closure of the posterior neuropore results in *myelomeningocele*. Complete failure of fusion along the entire length of the neural tube (*craniorachischisis*) usually results in early fetal death.

Following the birth of a child with a neural tube defect, the chance of anencephaly or myelomeningocele in a subsequent pregnancy is approximately 2%. After two affected fetuses, the risk of recurrence is almost 6%. Dietary supplementation of folic acid prior to and during the first six weeks of pregnancy reduces the risk of spina bifida. The same malformation is likely to repeat itself within a given family. Prenatal diagnosis is possible in every case by the combination of measuring the maternal serum concentration of α-fetoprotein and performing an ultrasound examination of the fetus. α-fetoprotein is the principal plasma protein of the fetus and is normally found in the amniotic fluid. Its concentration increases when the fetus has a skin defect such as anencephaly or myelomeningocele. α-fetoprotein is normally present in low concentrations in maternal serum but is elevated when the fetus has a neural tube defect.

Increased maternal folate intake before and during pregnancy markedly reduces the incidence of neural tube defects. Peri-conceptional supplementation of 4 mg of folic acid/day achieves a 70% reduction in neural tube defect recurrence and has similar benefits for first pregnancies. The fortification of flour with folic acid in the United States achieved a 19% national reduction in neural tube defects.

Anterior Neuropore Defects

Anencephaly   Anencephaly is a failure of the anterior neuropore to either close or remain closed at 24 days' gestation. The lamina terminalis does not form, and most of the forebrain does not develop. Because the forebrain is unformed, the neuroectoderm does not induce the overlying mesoderm to develop, the cranium, meninges, and scalp. The defect is worldwide in distribution and occurs in all ethnic groups, although with a higher incidence among Europeans than among Africans. The overall incidence of dysraphia is lowest in Orientals. Among this group, however, anterior cranial defects are relatively more common.

- **Clinical features.** Polyhydramnios is associated with less than 1% of normal births but with nearly 50% of anencephalic births. More than 50% of children with anencephaly are stillborn, and only 5% are alive at 7 days. The lamina terminalis fails to form and most forebrain structures do not develop. The deficient forebrain does not induce development of the overlying cranium, meninges, and scalp. Because a dermal covering is absent, hemorrhagic and fibrotic cerebral tissue, which lacks the appearance of normal brain, lies exposed to view. The optic nerves and the chiasm are usually intact, the hypothalamus is absent, and the anterior portion of the pituitary is usually present. All the endocrine organs are smaller than normal.

  The entire cranial vault is underdeveloped, resulting in hollow orbits and protruding eyes. Retroflexion of the neck is a common posture and may result from continuation of the cranial defect into the upper cervical segments. The arms, overgrown as compared with the legs, show the greatest disproportion in the proximal segments. The overall appearance of the anencephalic newborn is grotesque and described as *toad-like*. The face may show midline hypoplasia, similar to holoprosencephaly (Sarnat and Flores-Sarnat, 2001).
- **Diagnosis.** The prenatal diagnosis of anencephaly is possible as early as 12 weeks' gestation by measuring maternal serum concentrations of a-fetoprotein and by ultrasonography.
- **Management.** Make no effort to sustain life.

Encephalocele   An encephalocele is a protrusion of cortex and meninges, covered by skin, through a bony defect in the skull. Encephaloceles may occur in a frontal, nasopharyngeal, temporal, or parietal location, but most are located in the midline of the occipital bone. Frontal encephaloceles are more common in Southeast Asia. They nearly always include olfactory tissue. The incidence in the United States is 1 per 10,000 live births. Encephaloceles may occur in isolation or as part of a broader phenotype of single gene mutations.

- **Clinical features.** Encephaloceles vary in size from a small protrusion the diameter of a quarter to a sphere that equals the volume of the skull. The size of the sac does not indicate its contents. Some of the larger cysts contain only meninges and cerebrospinal fluid (CSF). Masses with a sessile base more often contain cerebral tissue than those that are pedunculated. Encephaloceles are rarely solitary defects. Rather, they tend to be associated with deformities of the cranial vault, absence or hypoplasia of the falx and tentorium, aplasia of the vermis of the cerebellum with deformity of the tectum, and disorganization of the underlying cerebral hemispheres. Despite its midline location, the derivation of the protruded material is usually from only one hemisphere. The hemisphere of origin is smaller than the normal contralateral hemisphere and displaced across the midline by the normal hemisphere. The ventricular system may be partially herniated into the encephalocele resulting in hydrocephalus.
- **Diagnosis.** MRI determines the contents of the sac.
- **Management.** The contents of the sac and the extent of associated anomalies help determine the usefulness of surgical intervention. The cerebral tissue within the sac is usually hamartomatous. The remaining intracranial brain may be dysplastic as well. Major surgery should be discouraged in the presence of generalized cerebral deformity. In such cases, some remedial procedure is usual for survivors to facilitate subsequent nursing care. Occipital meningoceles, although extremely large, may contain no neural tissue and amputation is possible. The long-term prognosis, although dependent on the concurrence of associated cerebral anomalies, is often favorable.

Posterior Neuropore Defects

The nomenclature used to describe defects of posterior neuropore closure is sufficiently bewildering to justify a review of definitions. *Spina bifida*, a midline separation of the vertebrae, is termed *occulta* if skin covers the defect. Spina bifida is commonly associated with neural disturbances, while spinal bifida occulta is usually asymptomatic and brought to attention only by incidental radiographs of the spine. The presence of abnormalities in the skin overlying a spina bifida occulta (such as an abnormal tuft of hair, pigmentation, a sinus opening, or a mass) is a malevolent sign that indicates an underlying defect of the neural tube.

Myeloschisis indicates that both the neural tube and its coverings are fully open. *Myelomeningocele* is the protrusion of a cystic mass of meninges, spinal cord, and CSF through a spina bifida; and *meningocele* is a cystic lesion composed only of meninges and spinal fluid without neural elements. *Myelodysplasia* is a malformation of the conus medullaris underlying, but not protruding through, a spinal bifida.

Myelomeningocele   Nonclosure of the posterior neuropore before 26 days of gestation causes spinal dysraphism. The mechanism by which closure fails is unexplained. It is not caused by increased pressure within the developing ventricular system since the choroid plexuses is not yet formed. Myelomeningocele is a combined malformation in the development of the neural tube and its mesodermal coverings. Although the severity of the disturbance in the neuroectoderm and the mesoderm usually is comparable, one may predominate or may exist as the sole feature of dysraphia.

- **Clinical features.** Most myelomeningoceles are lumbosacral in location, but some occur in the thoracic or cervical regions. The level of involvement determines much of the clinical deficit. The range of problems includes no deficit in the cases of *spina bifida occulta* without herniation of tissue and *mild spina bifida cystica* with herniation of meninges alone. More severe deficits accompany the herniation of nerve roots (meningomyelocele) and the parenchyma of the spinal cord (myelodysplasia). Hydrocephalus is a common complication, involving most patients with meningomyelocele and causing neurological deficit.

  Motor dysfunction results from interruption of the corticospinal tracts and from dysgenesis of the segmental innervation. At birth, the legs are flaccid and the hips dislocated. Spastic paraplegia, a spastic bladder, and a level of sensory loss develop in infants with a thoracic lesion (Table 8–1). At birth, clinical evidence of hydrocephalus is present in 15% of affected

TABLE 8–1   Clinical features of myelomeningocele

Motor function	Pathology	Sensory loss	Bladder function
Spastic paraplegia	Thoraco-lumbar	Sensory level present with segmental withdrawal reflex below	Spastic with automatic function
Flaccid paraplegia	Myeloschisis and myelodysplasia of the conus medullaris	Lumbosacral sensory loss with absence of withdrawal reflex	Flaccid, distended, overflow incontinence
Mixed paraplegia	Myeloschisis and myelody splasis of the conus medullaris	Sensory level with withdrawal reflexes	Spastic or flaccid depending on segment
Spastic monoplegia	Unilateral myeloschisis	Variable	Normal
Normal	Meningocele or myelodysplasia	None	Normal

newborns, but will eventually develop in 80%. Type II Chiari malformation is consistently present and aqueductal stenosis coexists in 50%.

Among newborns with a cystic protrusion, the sac is a meningocele in 10 to 20% and a myelomeningocele in the remainder. Sometimes, inspection differentiates meningoceles from myelomeningoceles. Meningoceles more often have a dermal covering fused to the underlying meninges, and tend to be pedunculated with the base forming a narrow channel connecting the sac to the spinal cord. The spinal cord underlying a meningocele is frequently deformed. Myelomeningoceles, by contrast, usually have a broad base and have only a partial epithelial covering. The dome oozes a combination of CSF and serum. Remnants of the spinal cord fuse to the exposed dorsal portion of the dome with the sac lying in a ventral position. Spinal roots and peripheral nerves originating from the involved segments of spinal cord traverse the cystic cavity in order to exit through their appropriate foramina. A variety of recognizable abnormalities of neuronal migration and prosencephalization are associated with myelomeningocele; these malformations are more critical to eventual intellectual outcome than is hydrocephalus (Table 8–2).

- **Diagnosis.** Prenatal diagnosis is accurate for diagnosis either by ultrasonography or by measuring a-fetoprotein concentrations in amniotic fluid (14–16 weeks' gestation) or maternal blood (16–18 weeks' gestation).
- **Management.** Delivery by cesarean section before the onset of labor may result in better subsequent motor development. After birth, the critical steps in formulating a management plan are (1) to determine the extent of neurological dysfunction caused by the myelopathy; (2) to assess the potential for hydrocephalus; and (3) to identify other malformations in the nervous system and visceral organs. When myelomeningocele is the only deformity, the newborn is alert and responsive and has no difficulty in feeding. Small defects are easily closed surgically in the neonatal period. Large defects that cause complete paraplegia and flaccid neurogenic bladder are associated with poor quality of life.

The immediate complications of large myelomeningoceles are hydrocephalus and infection from leaking CSF. Long-term complications include chronic urinary tract infections, decubiti, hydrocephalus, paraplegia, and other neurological deficits. Intrauterine surgery to close the back is an experimental procedure based on the hypotheses that exposure of the cord to amniotic fluid increases injury and increases hindbrain herniation (Tulipan et al., 1998). The usefulness of the procedure is not established.

TABLE 8.2   Adverse factors in myelomeningocele

1. No movement at knees or ankles
2. Clinical evidence of kyphosis or scoliosis
3. Congenital hydrocephalus with head circumference greater than the 95th percentile
4. Birth injury or asphyxia
5. Associated major birth defects

Spina Bifida Occulta *Spina bifida occulta* is an example of a predominantly mesodermal abnormality. The prominent bony change is the partial or complete absence of the vertebral arches with lateral displacement of the pedicles. Minor defects in the closure of the vertebral arches (defects covered by skin) are relatively common. Only in rare instances are they associated with a significant underlying deformity of the spinal cord. Scoliosis and kyphosis develop at the site of the bony abnormality when there is an underlying neural defect. While these conditions may be present at birth, they tend to become progressively severe with time. The more significant abnormalities of the cord are at its caudal extreme, where abnormal attachments may produce *a tethering effect*. A tethered cord is usually asymptomatic at birth but result in a traction injury to the cord and nerve roots as the child grows. The usual clinical features are disturbances of gait and sphincter control.

Diastematomyelia and Diplomyelia Diastematomyelia and diplomyelia are related malformations (Pang et al., 1992). Duplication of the spinal cord characterizes diplomyelia while two hemichords exist in diastematomyelia. The cord is normal in the cervical and upper thoracic regions and then divides into lateral halves for 1 to 10 segments. In diplomyelia, the separation is permanent. Each half of the cord is in its own sheath of dura mater separated by a septum composed of bone, cartilage, or fibrous tissue. In diastematomyelia, the separation is milder; both cords are within a single dural tube, no septum is present, and the two halves always rejoin caudally to form a single normal spinal cord.

The septum, which projects as a bony spur from the vertebral body, does not cause the split cord. Diastematomyelia occurs in the absence of a septum and is usually only one part of a larger dysraphic syndrome. Other associated anomalies are spina bifida occulta (or other vertebral abnormalities) and, in some cases, myelomeningocele. The essential fault in the development of diastematomyelia is the formation of more than one luminal border. Each border then induces a germinal matrix. The mechanism by which multiple luminal borders form is unknown. Several reports of familial occurrence suggest a genetic predisposition.

A report of two sisters with diastematomyelia suggests a genetic basis (Balci et al., 1999). All reported familial cases have been female suggesting X-linked dominant inheritance with lethality in hemizygous males.

- **Clinical features.** The onset of symptoms is anytime from birth to adult life. Among newborns, the presence of an abnormal tuft of hair over the spine or an associated meningoceles often brings the defect to attention.
- **Diagnosis.** MRI provides definitive visualization of the defect.
- **Management.** Surgical removal of the septum and general freeing of the cord from any tethering action helps prevent the further development of cord dysfunction.

Dermal Sinus These midline lesions result from an abnormal invagination of the ectoderm into the closure site of either the posterior or the anterior neuropore. Consequently, the sinus is always located in the lumbosacral or occipital region. Most sinuses terminate harmlessly in the subcutaneous tissue either as a blind pouch or as a dermoid cyst. Some extend to the neuraxis and serve as a portal by which infection may reach the CNS. These are usually associated with a spina bifida at the vertebral level corresponding to the dermatome at the opening in the skin and the spinal cord segment where the sinus terminates. The attachment of the sinus to the neuraxis may be epidural, intradural, or intramedullary. As the sinus approaches the dorsal surface of the spinal cord, it forms either a fibrous band or a dermoid cyst. The cyst acts as an expanding mass that compresses the underlying spinal cord.

Intracranial dermal sinuses, like their vertebral counterparts, either terminates as a harmless subcutaneous cyst or may extend through a defect in the occipital bone to reach the posterior fossa. Within the posterior fossa, the sinus usually expands into a cystic mass located either in the cerebellum or in the fourth ventricle.

- **Clinical features.** The opening in the skin over the spine is small. Ordinarily, it would escape attention, except that either a tuft of hair or a port wine stain usually marks the site. Intracranial dermal sinuses appear externally as a dimple in the skin overlying the external occipital protuberance.
- **Diagnosis.** The detection of a midline dermal orifice surrounded by a tuft of hair or a port-wine stain should lead to MRI of the underlying vertebrae or skull. The presence of a bony defect significantly increases the likelihood that the tract extends to the neuraxis and that it has the potential to produce infection or compression of the CNS. When meningitis occurs, Escherichia coli or *Staphylococcus aureus* is the organism most often identified as responsible, but in one-half of cases, the cultures are sterile. Investigate any child with midline dimple who develops meningitis or neurological dysfunction for a dermal sinus with the intention of surgically obliterating the tract or removing the cyst.

Lumbosacral Lipoma   Lipomas overlying the lumbosacral vertebrae, with or without an underlying spina bifida occulta, are usually harmless collections of subcutaneous fatty tissue. Some extend as a fibrous band that traverses the dura and then attach to the conus medullaris as an internal lipomatous mass. These extensions, not usually associated with other congenital anomalies, are *lipomeningoceles*.

- **Clinical features.** The subcutaneous lipoma is of variable size at birth and always well covered by skin. The lipomeningocele is asymptomatic at birth but tethers the cord; with time, the tether causes a progressive disturbance in gait and sphincter control.
- **Diagnosis.** All newborns with lumbosacral lipomas should have MRI of the spine.
- **Management.** Surgical removal of the lipoma and mobilization of the spinal cord is essential if the child shows evidence of a tethered cord.

The Chiari Malformation

Elongation of the cerebellar vermis with herniation of its caudal extreme through the foramen magnum is the essential feature of the Chiari malformation and called *Chiari type I*. Chiari type I is a common asymptomatic finding on magnetic resonance imaging (MRI) of the head and neck in older children and adults. *Chiari type II* is an additional downward displacement of a distorted lower medulla and dysplasia of medullary nuclei. It is a constant feature of lumbosacral myelomeningocele. *Chiari type III* is a rare malformation characterized by cervical spina bifida with cerebellar encephalocele. Hydrocephalus is an associated feature of types II and III. The herniated portions of the vermis may be necrotic from ischemia. Downward displacement of the cerebellum produces compression and kinking of the underlying medulla and upper cervical cord. The brainstem and fourth ventricle displace caudally and the cranial nerves arising in the medulla elongate in their course to the appropriate foramina.

- **Pathophysiology.** The pathogenesis of the Chiari malformation is not resolved, but a genetic basis is not established nor is downward traction from a tethered spinal cord responsible. Aplasia of the cerebellar vermis is common and the dentate and inferior olivary nuclei may be dysplastic. The hindbrain deformities initiate in fetuses of less than 20 weeks' gestation and probably become progressively severe as the brain grows during the second half of gestation. Development of the surrounding skull modifies by the need to accommodate the displaced contents of the posterior fossa. The foramen magnum enlarges, the clivus thins, and the posterior fossa diminishes in volume.
- **Clinical features.** Chiari I malformations are asymptomatic in newborns. Some may have abnormal control of breathing and eye movement disorders.
- **Diagnosis.** Head and neck MRI shows the low-lying cerebellar tonsils below the level of the foramen magnum.
- **Management.** Compromise of respiratory function requires decompression of the posterior fossa.

Ventral Dysraphia

Neuroenteric cyst is the only defect of the ventral surface of the neural tube that produces clinical manifestations in the newborn. The cyst derives from a fistula between the spinal cord and the gut or its derivatives. The fistula represents a failure in the complete separation of the primitive gut from the notochord. Neuroenteric cysts are most commonly located in the lower cervical and upper thoracic segments of the spine at the level where the primitive lung buds sprout from the foregut on the 25th day. On gross inspection, the cyst appears to be of neural origin because it attaches to the vertebrae, dura, or spinal cord. Microscopic examination of the cyst wall reveals a lining of non-ciliated columnar epithelial cells attached to a basement membrane and secrete mucin. Some portions of the cyst wall duplicate the layers of the intestinal tract completely.

- **Clinical features.** The presenting symptoms of neuroenteric cyst relate either to spinal cord compression or to meningitis. The onset of symptoms, is usually within the first six months, but may delay until adult life. Other anomalies of the nervous system, gastrointestinal tract, and heart may be associated.

- **Diagnosis.** Radiographs of the spine usually show dorsal or ventral spina bifida, hemivertebrae, fused vertebrae, or widening of the vertebral bodies. The definitive diagnosis relies on visualization of the cyst by MRI. Surgical extirpation of the mass relieves the spinal cord compression and provides a permanent cure.

Anterior Sacral Meningocele   This is an uncommon defect transmitted as an autosomal dominant trait (Lynch et al., 2000). It occurs more often in females and is associated with malformations of the reproductive organs. The bony abnormality is usually in the lower sacral or coccygeal region but not necessarily in the midline. An anterior sacral meningocele protrudes through a partial absence of the sacrum and coccyx. Symptoms included constipation and urinary incontinence. The meningocele presents as a mass in the abdominal cavity.

Caudal Regression Syndrome

The caudal regression syndrome is not a single entity but covers several malformations of the caudal spine. The extreme example is *sirenomelia*, in which only one leg is present. Although the name implies that the cord formed properly and then regressed, defects in neural tube closure and prosencephalization are often associated features. The risk of caudal regression is greater among infants of diabetic mothers. The clinical spectrum varies from absence of the lumbosacral spinal cord, resulting in small, paralyzed legs, to a single malformed leg associated with malformations of the rectum and genitourinary tract.

PROSENCEPHALIZATION

The neural tube is the anlage of the segmental nervous system from the midbrain to the sacrum. After the neural tube has formed and closed, the next stage in cerebral organogenesis is the development of suprasegmental structures: the cerebellum, the quadrageminal plate, and the forebrain.

Normal Prosencephalization

The forebrain (diencephalon and telencephalon) develops at 25 to 30 days' gestation from the rostral extent of the neural tube by the generation of a midline vesicle from the dorsal lip of the anterior neuropore. This midline vesicle is the primordium of the third ventricle and the foramina of Monro. Around it will develop the diencephalon and the rhinic lobe of the telencephalon. At 30 to 40 days, the cleavage and out pouching of the midline vesicle forms the bilateral cerebral vesicles. These will develop into those portions of the lateral ventricles, which, the limbic lobes surround at a future time. Finally, at 80 to 90 days, the lateral cerebral vesicles elaborate further into the complex tubular structures that will serve as the core of the supralimbic lobes. Therefore, the second and third months are the period when prosencephalization occurs.

This section discusses three major disturbances in prosencephalization. One is a defect, partial or complete, in the cleavage of the embryonic forebrain into two separate hemispheres. The second is a failure to establish commissural connections between the hemispheres, and the third is failure to develop optic nerves, septum pellucidum, and pituitary gland. The first two are frequently associated.

Defective Cleavage of the Forebrain

Following closure of the anterior neuropore, a rostral membrane is formed called the *lamina terminalis*. Disorders of the lamina terminalis lead first to midline defects and then to the disturbances of the forebrain. After differentiating the forebrain structures, the lamina terminalis becomes the anterior wall of the third ventricle. A malformation spectrum results from defective cleavage of the embryonic forebrain. The minimal anomaly, which serves as the common denominator for this group, is absence of the olfactory bulbs and tracts (*arhinencephaly*). Aplasia of the rhinic lobe may be associated but is not a constant feature. *Holotelencephaly* is a more severe defect in cleavage in which the third ventricle and diencephalic nuclei differentiate but the hemispheres do not. *Holoprosencephaly*, in which the two hemispheres are fused, is the most severe form (Table 8–3).

Arhinencephaly

Arhinencephaly is the absence of the olfactory bulbs and tracts. It often occurs in association with holoprosencephaly but may occur as a solitary malformation.

- **Clinical features.** Arhinencephaly without other forebrain malformations is associated with anosmia and lack of secretion of gonadotropic hormones

TABLE 8–3 Facial abnormalities associated with defects in prosencephalization

Severe
Medial monophthalmia (cyclopia), anophthalmia, microphthalmia
Absent, single, or double proboscis
Cleft lip and palate

Moderate
Hypotelorism, microphthalmia
Premaxillary agenesis, flat proboscis with single nostril
Cleft lip

Mild
Hypotelorism
Micrognathia
Cleft lip

(*Kallmann's syndrome*) (Gasztonyi et al., 2000). The syndrome is inherited as either an X-linked or autosomal dominant trait. Affected male newborns may have a small penis and cryptorchidism.

- **Diagnosis.** MRI shows the cerebral malformation. Lack of the postnatal rise of leuteinizing hormone and testosterone during infancy confirms hypogonadism.
- **Management.** Gonadotropic hormone replacement may restore fertility.

Holoprosencephaly

Holoprosencephaly (HPE) is a brain anomaly in which the forebrain fails to divide into two separate hemispheres and ventricles. A continuum of malformations are encompassed that include *alobar HPE* (a single ventricle and no separation of the cerebral hemispheres); *semilobar HPE* (fusion of the left and right frontal and parietal lobes with the interhemispheric fissure only present posteriorly); and lobar HPE (most of the right and left cerebral hemispheres and lateral ventricles are separated with fusion of the frontal lobes) (Muenke and Gropman, 2005).

Other central nervous system abnormalities not specific to HPE also occur. Olfactory and callosal agenesis is an almost constant feature of holoprosencephaly. Disrupted cerebral hemispheric organization results in heterotopic neurons and glial cells in the white matter and meninges, and disorganization of the cortical gray matter lamination.

- **Clinical features.** Midline facial abnormalities occur in 93% of newborns with holoprosencephaly. To some extent, the severity of the facial defect indicates the severity of the cerebral malformation. These range from hypotelorism to midline facial aplasias with fusion of the eyes (cyclops) and malformation and displacement of the nose. Malformations of the viscera and the musculoskeletal system occur in one-third. Seizures are common, often starting as infantile spasms. Severe development delay is the rule and hydrocephalus may be associated. Hypothalamic or pituitary dysfunction is present in infants with midline defects.
- **Diagnosis.** MRI accurately identifies the severity of the malformation. Approximately 25–50% of patients have chromosomal abnormality. Approximately 18–25% of patients with monogenic HPE have a recognizable syndrome. Several of the mutations causing nonsyndromic HPE are identifiable by molecular genetic testing. MRI imaging of the brain confirms the diagnosis of HPE, defines the anatomic subtype, and identifies associated CNS anomalies.
- **Management.** Treatment includes seizure control, correction of endocrine disturbances, and relief of hydrocephalus.

Septo-Optic Dysplasia

Septo-optic dysplasia is a clinically heterogeneous disorder defined by any combination of optic nerve hypoplasia, pituitary gland hypoplasia, and midline abnormalities of the brain. The combination of septo-optic dysplasia and absence of the corpus callosum and septum pellucidum is *DeMorsier syndrome*. Genetic transmission of familial cases is autosomal recessive and the abnormal gene location is *3p21.2–p21.1*. Midline defects of the septum pellucidum and hypothalamus may be associated. Other associated anomalies include midline cerebellar defects and hydrocephalus.

- **Clinical features.** Optic nerve hypoplasia may cause pendular nystagmus shortly after birth. Some males have micropenis and cryptorchidism. Hypoglycemia causes neonatal seizures. Mental retardation and epilepsy are common outcomes. The spectrum of congenital pituitary defects, range in severity from isolated growth hormone deficiency to panhypopituitarism (Thomas et al., 2001). When hypoplasia is severe, the child is severely visually impaired and the eyes draw attention because of strabismus and nystagmus. Ophthalmoscopic examination reveals a small, pale nerve head. A pigmented area surrounded by a yellowish mottled halo is sometimes present at the edge of the disk margin, giving the appearance of a double ring. The degree of hypothalamic–pituitary involvement varies. Possible symptoms include neonatal hypoglycemia and seizures, recurrent hypoglycemia in childhood, growth retardation, diabetes insipidus, and sexual infantilism. Some combination of mental retardation, cerebral palsy, and epilepsy is often present and indicates malformations in other portions of the brain.
- **Diagnosis.** Required studies in all infants with ophthalmoscopic evidence of optic nerve hypoplasia are MRI of the head and assessment of endocrine function. The common findings on MRI are cavum septum pellucidum, hypoplasia of the cerebellum, aplasia of the corpus callosum, aplasia of the fornix, and an empty sella. Endocrine studies include assays of growth hormone, antidiuretic hormone, and the integrity of hypothalamic–pituitary control of the thyroid, adrenal, and gonadal systems. Infants with hypoglycemia usually have growth hormone deficiency.
- **Management.** The endocrine abnormalities respond to replacement therapy.

Colpocephaly

Colpocephaly is a selective dilatation of the occipital horns caused by loss of the surrounding white matter. Intraventricular pressure is not increased. It occurs as a primary malformation in association with a poorly laminated striate cortex, subcortical heterotopia, and defective ependyma lining the occipital horns, with migrational defects or agenesis of the corpus callosum, and secondary to periventricular leukomalacia, especially in premature infants, because of loss of periventricular white matter in the posterior half of the cerebral hemispheres.

- **Clinical features.** The child may appear normal at birth but mental retardation, spastic diplegia, epilepsy, and vision loss are all possible outcomes. Some infants come to attention because of an enlarging head circumference.

- **Diagnosis.** MRI shows the posterior ventricular enlargement and other associated malformations.
- **Management.** Seizures treatment is often required. Shunting is not required because the intraventricular pressure is normal.

Agenesis of the Corpus Callosum

Anomalous development of the three-telencephalic commissures, the corpus callosum, the anterior commissure, and the hippocampal commissure, is relatively common. All three commissures develop from the anlage of the telencephalon at the site of its junction with the diencephalon. This junctional region divides into a ventral *lamina terminalis* and a dorsal *lamina reuniens*. The commissures derive, between 40 and 80 days' gestation, from a local thickening of the lamina terminalis called the commissural plate. The commissural plate serves as a bridge for axonal passage. Without this plate, the corpus callosum cannot form.

The prevalence of agenesis of the corpus callosum is 2% in North America and 8% in Japan. Most are isolated malformations, but callosal agenesis also occurs as part of several syndromes. Associated anomalies are aplasia of the cerebellar vermis and anomalous pyramidal tract formation. Callosal agenesis may involve the entire commissure; when partial, the splenium is the part usually lacking. Partial agenesis is more common than total agenesis. The minimal defect is a thinning of the splenium in association with enlargement of the occipital horns. In callosal agenesis, the anterior and hippocampal commissures are always well formed or large.

Callosal agenesis is an additional feature of many other prosencephalic dysplasias. It occurs with aplasia of the cerebellar vermis and anomalous pyramidal tract formation. Without the restraining forces of the callosal fibers, the roof of the third ventricle rises to a dorsal position and the foramina of Monro greatly enlarge. The result is a single 'bat-shaped' vesicle formed by the third and lateral ventricles. The septi pellucidi appear to be absent, but in fact, they lie in an almost horizontal position between the fornix and Probst's bundle. The cingulate gyrus is normal in size but has a simplified convolutional pattern.

- **Clinical features.** Callosal agenesis in the absence of other brain malformations is not detectable by ordinary neurological examination. Specialized testing is required to show deficits in the interhemispheric transfer of perceptual information for verbal expression. Mental retardation or learning disabilities occur in some cases. Seizures, when they occur, are probably secondary to minor focal cortical dysplasias. Hypertelorism is often present and may be associated with exotropia and inability to converge. The onset of seizures varies from the day of birth to three months postpartum. Neonatal apnea is common. The apnea progresses to generalized seizures and flexion spasms. The combination of infantile spasms and agenesis of the corpus callosum is *Aicardi syndrome*. Ocular malformations may be associated. The syndrome occurs almost exclusively in females, and X-linked inheritance with male lethality is a possible mechanism.

The syndrome most often encountered in newborns that survive to infancy is megalencephaly and developmental delay. Head circumference increases to just above the 98th percentile and then parallels the normal growth curve. These children show mild developmental delay and have borderline intelligence as adults. The mental impairment is probably due to neuronal disorganization in the cortex.

- **Diagnosis.** Computed tomography (CT), often performed because of the suspicion of hydrocephalus, reveals the characteristic ventricular configuration of agenesis of the corpus callosum. The lateral ventricles are widely separated, the occipital horns relatively dilated, and the third ventricle sits between the lateral ventricles. A characteristic EEG pattern is interhemispheric asynchrony, especially of sleep spindles. In *Aicardi syndrome*, a burst suppression pattern arises independently and asynchronously from the two hemispheres.
- **Management.** Treatment is supportive, anticonvulsant therapy and special education.

HISTOGENESIS

The events of neural maturation after initial induction and formation of the neural tube are each predictive of specific types of malformation of the brain and of later abnormal neurological function. These are (1) mitotic proliferation of neuroblasts; (2) programmed death of excess neuroblasts; (3) neuroblast migration; (4) growth of axons and dendrites; (5) electrical polarity of the cell membrane; (6) synaptogenesis; (7) biosynthesis of neurotransmitters; and (8) myelination of axons.

The bulk growth of the cerebral hemispheres is slow, but steady at 2 to 6 months and then accelerates during the last trimester. At the beginning of the second month, the cytoarchitecture of the hemispheres is divisible into four layers. Innermost is a two-layered germinal matrix. Separated from the germinal matrix is the third layer: a primitive stratum of pyramidal cells. The outermost fourth layer is relatively clear of cells and termed *the layer of His*. Successive waves of neurons migrate to the surface of the cerebral hemispheres in the ensuing months. New cellular layers form from within outward. It is not until the sixth month that a six-layered neocortex is recognizable. At 10 to 15 weeks, the first hemispheric fissures appear and the smooth exterior of the forebrain converts into the pattern of gyri and sulci that will bury 75% of the cortical surface (Table 8–4).

Disorders of Early Neuronal Migration (8–20 Weeks' Gestation)

Destructive processes, especially those that persist for extended periods, or an inadequate mitotic proliferation of neuroblasts causes cerebral hypoplasia. The entire brain may be affected, or portions may be selectively involved. Cerebellar hypoplasia is often a selective interference with proliferation of the external granular layer.

TABLE 8–4   Development of the cerebral sulci and fissures

10 to 15 weeks
Interhemispheric fissure
Sylvian fissure
Transverse cerebral fissure
Callosal sulcus

16 to 19 weeks
Parieto-occipital fissure
Olfactory sulcus
Cingulate sulcus
Calcerine fissure

20 to 23 weeks
Rolandic sulcus
Superior temporal sulcus

24 to 27 weeks
Prerolandic sulcus
Middle temporal sulcus
Postrolandic sulcus
Superior frontal sulcus

28 to 31 weeks
Inferior temporal sulcus
Inferior frontal sulcus

32 to 35 weeks
Secondary sulci completed

36 to 40 weeks
Tertiary sulci completed

Lissencephaly (Agyria) and Subcortical Band Heterotopia

Lissencephaly encompasses several disorders of neuronal migration in which neurons destined to form the superficial layers of the cerebral cortex fail to complete their journey (Kato and Dobyns, 2003). Neuroblasts that never migrate from the periventricular region form *periventricular nodular heterotopia*. This is an X-linked genetic disorder secondary to defective expression of the gene *Filamin-1*. Neuroblasts that migrate only to the subcortical white matter form *subcortical laminar heterotopia*. Transmission is also X-linked but due to the gene *Doublecortin* (*DCX*). When neuroblasts reach the cortical plate but fail to form correct lamination, the cortical plate shows abnormal gyration (*lissencephaly*). Mutations in X-linked lissencephaly genes cause lissencephaly in hemizygous males and a milder phenotype, (*subcortical band heterotopia*) in females. The cortex lacks its normal convolutional pattern and nests of neurons accumulate in the white matter (*heterotopia*). Complete absence of gyri causes a smooth cerebral surface (*agyria*), while incomplete gyral formation causes a reduced number of convolutions that are large in size (*pachygyria*). Four major groups of lissencephaly exist: (1) the agyria-pachygyria-band spectrum with subcortical band heterotopia; (2) lissencephaly with other anomalies such as agenesis of the corpus callosum and cerebellar hypoplasia; (3) cobblestone dysplasia; and (4) microlissencephaly.

The agyria-pachygyria-band spectrum is the most common type of lissencephaly. Associated features are enlarged ventricles and a hypoplastic corpus callosum. The brainstem and cerebellum are usually normal.

In at least three disorders, migrational disturbances coexist with congenital muscular dystrophy. These are *Fukuyama CMD* (FCMD), *muscle–eye–brain disease* (MEBD), and the *Walker–Warburg syndrome* (WWS). FCMD occurs almost exclusively in Japan, MEBD occurs mainly in Finland, and WWS has wide geographical distribution. Each has a different gene abnormality.

- **Clinical features.** Some newborns have normal head circumference at birth but all will eventually have microcephaly. Minor facial abnormalities are constant features of newborns with agyria. The clinical features of *the Miller–Dieker syndrome* are microcephaly and a peculiar facies that includes micrognathia, high forehead, thin upper lip, short nose with anteverted nares, and low-set ears. Hypotonia is present at birth. In infancy, development is slow, hypotonia changes to spasticity, and intractable seizures are the rule. Most do not survive the first year.
- **Diagnosis.** MRI is the imaging study of choice. Chromosome and molecular diagnosis are available.
- **Management.** Management is symptomatic. Genetic counseling is available for many families.

Disturbances of Late Neuroblast Migration (After 20 Weeks' Gestation)

Neuronal migration continues after 20 weeks' gestation. Perinatal disorders, especially in the premature, may interfere with this process.

Disorders of Cerebellar Development

The cerebellum begins its phase of accelerated growth during the fifth month and continues to increase rapidly in volume through the first month postpartum. It derives from the alar plate of the rhombencephalon during the second month. The first portions of the cerebellum to differentiate are the flocculus and nodulus. They lie within the fourth ventricle at the level of the vestibular nuclei. The newer portions of the cerebellum form during the third month. Purkinje cells and large neurons of the deep nuclei are the first cells to reach their final position. Neuroblasts, originating in the rhombic lip, then migrate over the entire surface of the dorsal cerebellum to form the external granular layer. The cells of the external granular layer begin their inward migration at 30 weeks. They differentiate into small neurons and glia. The process of inward migration completes during infancy and abolishes the external granular layer.

The prolonged interval of neuroblast migration makes the cerebellum particularly vulnerable to perinatal and postnatal exposure to toxic effects of drugs, infections, and hypoxic-ischemic injuries. Complete agenesis of the cerebellum is unusual. More often, there is aplasia of one or more parts.

Agenesis of the Cerebellar Vermis   Aplasia of the vermis is relatively common and often associated with other cerebral malformations. All or part of the vermis may be missing, and when the vermis is incomplete, the caudal portion is usually lacking. Dominantly inherited aplasia of the anterior vermis is a rare condition.

- **Clinical features.** Partial agenesis of the cerebellar vermis may be asymptomatic. Symptoms are nonprogressive and vary from only mild gait ataxia and upbeating nystagmus to severe ataxia.

    Complete agenesis causes titubation of the head and truncal ataxia. Vermal agenesis is frequently associated with other cerebral malformations, producing a constellation of symptoms and signs referable to neurological dysfunction. Two such examples are the Dandy–Walker malformation (see Ch. 18) and the *Joubert syndrome.*

    The Joubert syndrome consists of four recessively inherited syndromes characterized by a characteristic facies, oculomotor apraxia, and hyperpnea intermixed with central apnea in the neonatal period (Valente et al., 2005). One of the phenotypes includes malformations in several viscera. Cerebellar vermal agenesis is a constant feature of the Joubert syndrome, but several other cerebral malformations are usually present as well. All patients are mentally retarded, and some are microcephalic. Several affected children have died unexpectedly, possibly from respiratory failure.
- **Diagnosis.** MRI shows agenesis of the vermis of the cerebellum with enlargement of the cisterna magna. Other cerebral malformations, such as agenesis of the corpus callosum, are also associated.

Agenesis of the Cerebellar Hemispheres   Congenital hypoplasia of the cerebellar hemispheres can be unilateral or bilateral. Unilateral cerebellar hypoplasia is not associated with genetic disorders, but more than half of patients with bilateral disease have an identifiable genetic disorder transmitted by autosomal recessive inheritance. Some families with cerebellar hemispheric and vermal hypoplasia have a genetic defect that maps to the short arm of the X-chromosome (Bertorini, 2000).

The common histological feature is the absence of granular cells, with relative preservation of Purkinje cells. In some hereditary forms, granular cell degeneration may continue postnatally and cause progressive cerebellar dysfunction during infancy.

- **Clinical features.** Cerebellar aplasia is generally asymptomatic in the newborn unless there are associated cerebral anomalies. Most will develop hypotonia, delayed development, truncal titubation, intention tremor, and fixation nystagmus during infancy.
- **Diagnosis.** MRI accurately identifies the portions of the cerebellum that are malformed as well as associated malformations.
- **Management.** Management is symptomatic.

Microcephaly Vera

Undergrowth of the brain and skull is a common consequence of brain damage from environmental agents. When damage occurs early in pregnancy, cerebral growth failure is already demonstrable at the time of birth. This helps establish the antepartum timing of brain damage since intrapartum brain damage will not produce a recognizable decrease in head circumference until 3 to 6 months postpartum.

After excluding microcephaly secondary to antepartum brain damage, a group of newborns remains with decreased head circumference at birth due to genetic or chromosomal disturbances (Battaglia and Carey, 2003). The cause of one form (MCPH1) is a mutation in the gene encoding *microcephalin* on chromosome 8p. Amish lethal microcephaly (*DNC* or *MUP1*) only occurs in old order Amish communities.

- **Clinical features.** Head circumference is less than 3%. Neurological examination is normal except for mental retardation. No skeletal or organ malformations are present. Mental retardation is severe when transmission is by autosomal recessive inheritance, but intelligence may be normal in families with autosomal dominant transmission. Newborns with microcephaly vera may have a characteristic appearance of the head: a disproportion exists between the size of the face and skull. The reduced size of the cranial vault causes thickening of the overlying scalp, which tends to cause deep folding in the occipital region.
- **Diagnosis.** MRI shows that the cerebral hemispheres are small, due to reduction in size of the cortex, which has a simplified convolutional pattern.
- **Management.** Treatment is supportive.

REFERENCES

Balci S, Caglar K and Eryilmaz, M. Diastematomyelia in two sisters. Am J Med Genet 1999;86:180–182.

Battaglia A and Carey JC. Microcephaly. In: CD Rudolph and AM Rudolph (eds). Rudolph's Pediatrics, 21st edn. London: McGraw-Hill, Chapter 10.4.3, 2003; pp. 784–786.

Bertorini E, des Portes V, Zanni G, et al. X-linked congenital ataxia: a clinical and genetic study. Am. J Med Genet 2000;92:53–56.

Gasztonyi Z, Barsi P and Czeizel AE. Kallmann syndrome in three unrelated women and an association with femur-fibula-ulna dysostosis in one case. Am J Med Genet. 2000;93:176–180.

Honein MA, Paulozzi LJ, Mathews TJ, et al. Impact of folic acid fortification of the US food supply on the occurrence of neural tube defects. JAMA 2001;285:2981–2986.

Kato M and Dobyns WB. Lissencephaly and the molecular basis of neuronal migration. Hum Molec Genet 2003;12(R1):R89–R96.

Kelley RI, Robinson D, Puffenberger EG, et al. Amish lethal microcephaly: A new metabolic disorder with severe congenital microcephaly and 2-ketoglutaric aciduria. Am J Med Genet 2002;112:318–326.

Lynch, SA, Wang Y, Strachan T, et al. Autosomal dominant sacral agenesis: Currarino syndrome. J Med Genet 2000;37:561–566.

Muenke M and Gropman A. Holoprosencephaly Overview. (Updated 11 March 2005) In: GeneClinics; Medical Genetic Knowledge Base. [database online] University of Washington, Seattle. Available at http://www.geneclinics.org

Sarnat HB and Flores-Sarnat L. Neuropathological research strategies in holoprosencephaly. J Child Neurol 2001;16:918–931.

Pang D, Dias MS and Ahab-Barmada M. Split cord malformation; Part 1: A unified theory of embryogenesis for double cord malformations. J Neurosurg 1992;31:481–500.

Thomas, PQ, Dattani MT, Brickman JM, et al. Heterozygous HESX1 mutations associated with isolated congenital pituitary hypoplasia and septo-optic dysplasia. Hum Mol Genet 2001;10:39–45.

Valente EM, Marsh SE, Castori M, et al. Distinguishing the four genetic causes of Joberts syndrome-related disorders. Ann Neurol 2005;57:513–519.

Wallis D and Muenke M. Mutations in holoprosencephaly. Hum Mutat 2000;16:99–108.

9

Hydrocephalus and Congenital Tumors

Gerald M. Fenichel

HYDROCEPHALUS

Several previous chapters discussed hydrocephalus as an accompanying feature of intracranial hemorrhage (Ch. 5), intrauterine infection (Ch. 6), and disorders of cerebral morphogenesis (Ch. 8). This section deals with those disorders in which neonatal hydrocephalus is the presenting and prominent manifestation of disease. Malformation of the ventricular system, in one or more places, is the common mechanism of the hydrocephalus.

Developmental Disorders of the Ventricular System

The Dandy–Walker Malformation

The essential components of the Dandy–Walker malformation are cystic dilation of the fourth ventricle and agenesis, or hypoplasia, of the cerebellar vermis. Often associated with the malformation is non-opening of the foramen of Magendie. Other features include cerebellar aplasia, heterotopia of the inferior olivary nuclei and pachygyria of the cerebral cortex (Fig. 9–1).

Atresia of the foramina of Magendie and Luschka, once considered the initiating feature of cyst formation, is not a constant feature. Furthermore, intrauterine stenosis of the foramina secondary to reactive gliosis does not reproduce the typical pathological features. Instead generalized ventricular dilation without either cyst formation or hypoplasia of the cerebellar vermis occurs. Other malformations of the brain are associated in two-thirds of

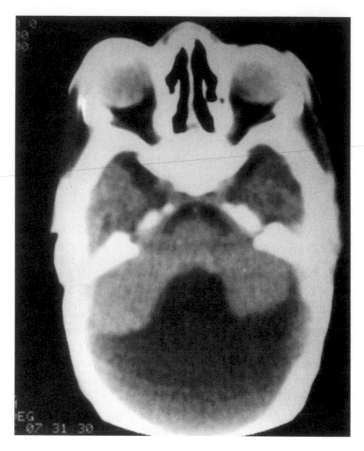

FIGURE 9–1   Dandy–Walker malformation. An enlarged cyst replacing the fourth ventricle as visualized by axial computed tomography. The vermis is hypoplastic.

cases. Most common is agenesis of the corpus callosum. Other malformations include heterotopia, abnormalities of gyral formation, dysraphic states, aqueductal stenosis, and congenital tumors. Facial angiomas, cardiovascular malformations, cleft palate, and ocular deformities are associated features in up to 10%. This suggests that the timing of the malformation is during the third and fourth gestational week.

The mechanism of the Dandy–Walker malformation remains uncertain. Possible causes include atresia of the foramen of Magendie and failure of the rhombic lips to differentiate fully from the roof of the rhombencephalon. A disturbance in cellular proliferation and migration of neurons from the rhombic lips of the alar plate could result in aplasia of the cerebellar vermis and in heterotopia of the inferior olive. Genetic causes are also possible. In one family, two sisters had three male fetuses with isolated Dandy–Walker variant (Wakeling et al., 2002).

- **Clinical features.** Prenatal hydrocephalus is not an obligatory feature. The onset of hydrocephalus, although variable, is usually within three months of birth. The cause of neurological handicaps, such as spastic diplegia and mental retardation, is more probably the associated cerebral malformations than the hydrocephalus. Bulging of the skull is more prominent in the occipital than in the frontal region. Neurological dysfunction, when present in the newborn, is referable to compression of structures within the posterior fossa: apneic spells, nystagmus, truncal ataxia, cranial nerve palsies, and hyperreflexia in the legs. The rapidity of head growth and ultimate head size are generally less severe than encountered with aqueductal stenosis or with the Chiari malformation. The combination of agenesis of the corpus callosum, the Dandy–Walker malformation, and hemimeganencephaly occurs in the *sebaceous nevus syndrome* (Dodge and Dobyns, 1995). The term encompasses several disorders.
- **Diagnosis.** MRI reveals cystic enlargement of the fourth ventricle and hypoplasia of the vermis. Upward displacement of the tentorium, torcula, straight sinus, and vein of Galen are associated features.
- **Management.** Shunting of the lateral ventricle alone provides immediate relief of hydrocephalus but fails to prevent delayed brainstem compression due to a buildup of pressure in the fourth ventricle. The procedure of choice is a dual shunt of both the lateral ventricle and the posterior fossa cyst. Children with shunts may develop symptoms that suggest shunt failure: lethargy, personality change, and vomiting. These episodes are transitory and often occur when the shunt is clearly patent. The mechanism of such episodes is unknown.

Aqueductal Stenosis

Obstruction of the cerebral aqueduct is the most common cause of congenital hydrocephalus. At birth, the mean length of the cerebral aqueduct is 12.8 mm. It narrows to its smallest diameter in the segment closest to the third ventricle, dilates in its central segment, and then narrows again before opening into the fourth ventricle. At its smallest cross-sectional diameter, the cerebral aqueduct of normal newborns is generally $0.5 \, \text{mm}^2$, and is always larger than $0.1 \, \text{mm}^2$. The small lumen of the cerebral aqueduct, in relationship to its length, makes it especially vulnerable to internal compromise from reactive gliosis and hemorrhage and external compression from tumors and venous malformations.

Infection, Chiari II malformation, and tumor are possible causes of congenital aqueductal stenosis. Chiari II malformation is the most common cause. Fourth ventricular enlargement is not a feature of solitary congenital stenosis. Such cases are usually sporadic, but five percent of all cases of congenital aqueduct stenosis are attributable to an X-linked form (Havercamp et al., 1999).

With the exception of X-linked aqueductal stenosis, most cases of congenital aqueductal stenosis show some degree of malformation or gliosis, or both. The presence of malformation (forking) of the cerebral aqueduct and the absence of gliosis may be related to the timing of the insult, prior to aqueductal formation, rather than to the cause. Gliosis does not occur in X-linked aqueductal stenosis. Instead, reduplication and heaping up of the ependymal lining are the common findings. Forking of the aqueduct also occurs. Whatever the underlying mechanism, obstruction of the cerebral aqueduct ultimately leads to dilation of the third and lateral ventricles. The thalami become widely separated, the septum pallucidum and the corpus callosum thinned and eventually destroyed, and the cerebral hemispheres compressed. Because the unmyelinated brain is especially compressible and the skull is distensible, there is little resistance to progressive dilation of the ventricles. Rupture of the ependymal lining of the lateral ventricle causes the CSF to dissect the cerebral parenchyma and to form a porencephalic cyst. Uninhibited dilation of the ventricular system eventually destroys the forebrain and results in hydranencephaly.

- **Clinical features.** Hydrocephalus is present at birth and detectable prenatally by ultrasound. The enlarged head circumference may result in cephalopelvic disproportion and poor progress of labor. The forehead is bowed, the scalp veins dilated, the sutures split, and the fontanelles increased in size and tension. These signs exaggerate when the child cries but fail to disappear even in the quiet state. A setting sun sign and abducens palsies may be present.
- **Diagnosis.** Prenatal diagnosis by ultrasound is the rule. Other abnormalities, usually spina bifida, are associated in more than 70% of cases. Postpartum, MRI readily accomplishes the diagnosis of aqueductal stenosis and visualizes associated malformations.
- **Management.** Congenital hydrocephalus secondary to aqueductal stenosis is severe, does not respond to medical therapy directed at decreasing the volume of CSF, nor does it arrest at a stage that is less than harmful to the brain. Diversion of the CSF from the ventricular system to an extracranial site by surgical shunting is the only effective method of management. Early delivery is the rule; balancing the risks of prematurity against progressive increased intracranial pressure. Initiate ventricular shunting promptly, but recognize that relief of hydrocephalus does not necessarily equate to a normal child. Early hydrocephalus, even when shunted, is frequently associated with mental retardation, motor deficits, and seizures.

X-linked Hydrocephalus (L1 Syndrome)   A mutation at gene site Xq28 causes the syndrome (Schandler-Stumpell and Vos, 2004). The gene encodes the L1 cell adhesion molecule (L1CAM).

- **Clinical features.** The onset of severe hydrocephalus is often before birth. Increased intraventricular fluid volume causes an increased occipital-frontal circumference. The occipital frontal circumference continues to grow rapidly after birth. Tendon reflexes are brisk. Other features of the X-linked phenotype include enlarged cerebral ventricles, mental retardation, spastic paraparesis, and adducted thumbs. The most severe cases die pre- or perinatally from severe hydrocephalus.
- **Diagnosis.** MRI shows increased ventricular size, loss of cerebral sulci, and transependymal resorption of cerebrospinal fluid. Bilateral absence of the pyramids is the rule. Molecular genetic testing of the L1CAM gene is available.
- **Management.** Treatment options are similar to those used for other forms of congenital hydrocephalus.

CONGENITAL TUMORS

The term *congenital tumor* encompasses both tumors derived from embryonic tissue and tumors presumed to have originated in utero. All tumors of childhood and some of adult life fit this definition. However, in keeping with the format previously established for this text, the discussion is limited to those tumors symptomatic in the newborn period.

Congenital Brain Tumors

Brain tumors that are symptomatic during the first two months usually have somewhat different histological and clinical features than those that become symptomatic during infancy (Fort and Rushing, 1997). The most common types are teratomas and neuroepithelial tumors (choroid plexus papillomas, astrocytomas, medulloblastomas, and ependymomas). Two-thirds are supratentorial in location and one-third infratentorial. Teratomas are usually supratentorial in location while only 30% of neuroepithelial tumors have a supratentorial location.

One possible clue to the pathogenesis of congenital brain tumors is the relative concurrence of tumors and malformations. Neurocutaneous syndromes epitomize this concurrence. Because tumor formation and malformation are both disorders of cellular proliferation, a noxious agent, if active during early embryogenesis, might stimulate either or both abnormalities. The relative oncogenicity or teratogenicity of a particular noxious agent might depend upon the virulence of the agent, the timing of the insult, the duration of exposure, and the genetic background and health of the embryo.

Astrocytoma

- **Clinical features.** Newborns with hemispheric gliomas either have intrauterine hydrocephalus producing cephalopelvic disproportion and dystocia, or develop hydrocephalus in the first days or weeks postpartum. The clinical features are those of increasing intracranial pressure: enlarging head size, separation of the sutures, lethargy, irritability, failure to feed, and vomiting. Seizures are uncommon and indicate that the tumor has hemorrhaged. Because some degree of hemorrhage occurs in and around most glial tumors, the cerebrospinal fluid usually contains blood or is xanthochromic in appearance.
- **Management.** In most newborns with hemispheric astrocytoma, CT performed for the evaluation of hydrocephalus accomplishes the diagnosis. Surgical extirpation of the tumor is rarely attempted. The outcome without surgery is poor and all have died.

Congenital glioma of the brainstem, like glioma of the brainstem in older children, causes dysfunction of brainstem nuclei without hydrocephalus. Recurrent episodes of apnea and tremors of the limbs mark the subsequent course. Death occurs in the first month.

Choroid Plexus Papilloma

Tumors of the choroid plexus occur, almost exclusively, during the first decade. They are generally benign but may be malignant and are usually located within one lateral ventricle. Of all neonatal tumors, benign choroid plexus papilloma has the best outcome. Surgical removal is possible.

- **Clinical features.** Papillomas produce a communicating hydrocephalus by the excessive secretion of CSF and may produce noncommunicating hydrocephalus as well by obstructing the foramen of Monro. Increased intracranial pressure accounts for the clinical features of enlarging head size, lethargy, and difficulty in feeding. Focal neurological deficits are uncommon. CSF pressure is very high, but the protein concentration is only mildly elevated, and xanthocromia is not present.
- **Diagnosis.** MRI shows an intraventricular enhancing mass with a peculiar 'cauliflower' shape. They are large, partially calcified, have a lobulated papillomatous appearance, and enhance homogeneously. The differential diagnosis of intraventricular tumors includes ependymoma and hemangioma. Ependymoma, a more common tumor of childhood than choroid plexus papilloma, is unusual in newborns. Ependymomas cause an obstructive hydrocephalus but do not increase the production of CSF. Hemangiomas of the choroid plexus can stimulate excessive production of cerebrospinal fluid, but are exceptionally rare in newborns.
- **Management.** The primary treatment objective for both low-grade and high-grade choroid plexus tumors is gross total resection. For choroid plexus papilloma, this is a curative procedure.

The major obstacle to the surgical removal of choroid plexus tumors is their rich vascular network within these tumors. The choroid plexus receives its blood supply from the anterior and posterior choroidal arteries, branches of the internal carotid artery and the posterior cerebral artery. The extent of surgical resection is the single most important factor that determines the prognosis of choroid plexus papilloma.

Medulloblastoma

Medulloblastoma is a primitive neuroectodermal tumor (PNET). Rare genetic syndromes predispose to medulloblastoma (Turcot, Gorlin, and Li–Fraumeni). Familial cases also occur that are unrelated to these syndromes (von Koch et al. 2002). Tumors have occurred in identical twins and in newborn siblings born at different times. *Trilateral retinoblastoma* is a familial syndrome with bilateral retinoblastomas and a pineoblastoma with retinoblastic features (Finelli et al., 1995).

- **Clinical features.** A relatively high incidence of stillbirth, hydrocephalus, and congenital malformation occurs among siblings of newborns with medulloblastoma. Newborns with medulloblastoma have a higher than usual incidence of malformations in other organs.

Tumors that produce clinical signs in the newborn already occupy large portions of the posterior fossa. The onset of oncogenesis, in such tumors, is probably early in embryogenesis. An enlarged head and tenseness of the fontanelle are constant signs; obstruction of the cerebral aqueduct by tumor causes dilation of the third and lateral ventricles. When the onset of symptoms is insidious, the first manifestation is difficulty in feeding. Lethargy, vomiting, and apnea accompany the increasing intracranial pressure. Nystagmus, downward tonic deviation of the eyes, and opisthotonus may be associated; seizures occur as well. Apnea, from compression of the brainstem, is the usual terminal event.

- **Diagnosis.** A contrast-enhanced brain MRI typically shows a heterogeneously enhancing mass in the fourth ventricle with obstructive hydrocephalus.
- **Management.** Death is invariable.

Meningeal Sarcoma

Malignant mesenchymal tumors of the meninges arise from primitive mesenchymal cells that surround the neural tube to form the dura. These cells are multipotential and may differentiate into several different tumor types.

- **Clinical features.** The initial features may be those of an intracranial mass, an occipital swelling, or cord compression. Intracranial sarcomas may be located either supra- or infratentorial. Most meningeal sarcomas present with hydrocephalus, much like other intracranial tumors, and rapidly lead to death. A few present as a swelling in the occipital region, that can be mistaken for either an encephalocele or a leptomeningeal cyst. The tumors, which are extradural in position, erode through the parietal and occipital bones. They are vascularized by the external carotid circulation. With room to grow extracranially, the mass can attain a large size.
- **Diagnosis.** Neuroimaging differentiates meningeal sarcoma from encephalocele and leptomeningocele cyst. The sarcoma is a solid tumor, outside the dura, that compresses the underlying brain.
- **Treatment.** Surgical extirpation has been successful in several cases. Radiation therapy is not beneficial.

Teratoma

Teratomas arise from primitive germinal cells. The mass usually contains a variety of tissue types. They tend to be located in the midline, usually in the pineal region. Other malignant tumors arising in this location include pineoblastoma and pineocytoma.

- **Clinical features.** Hydrocephalus is a constant feature of intracranial teratomas. In live births with small tumors, their midline position obstructs the cerebral aqueduct, and hydrocephalus develops during the first week. Live births with larger tumors have large heads at birth making vaginal delivery difficult because of cephalopelvic disproportion. Cranial nerve dysfunction and apnea are frequently associated. The largest tumors lead to intrauterine death. Tumor replaces much of the brain, and hydrocephalus is present as well.

- **Diagnosis.** Neuroimaging readily identifies the tumor size and location. Germ cell tumors typically show homogeneous enhancement with peripheral calcification on contrast-enhanced cranial MRI.
- **Treatment.** Attempts at surgical extirpation are rarely successful.

Congenital Spinal Cord Tumors

Neuroblastoma and teratoma are the only spinal cord tumors that occur with any frequency in the newborn.

Neuroblastoma

Neuroblastoma is the most common solid tumor of the newborn. Although one-half of cases occur during the first 2 years, the tumor is rarely symptomatic at birth. Neuroblastoma is a derivative of sympathetic neuroblasts of the neural crest, the anlage of the sympathetic ganglia, and therefore arises in many body sites. Prognosis depends upon tumor location and age at onset. Neuroblastomas of the thorax and mediastinum have the best prognosis. Children who manifest symptoms before the age of 1 year respond well to therapy and have spontaneous remissions; those who manifest symptoms after the age of 3 years respond poorly to therapy and are frequently dead within 2 years. Neuroblastoma in the newborn is frequently widespread at the time of birth and most die despite aggressive therapy. In those with spinal cord compression, neurological sequelae may persist even after complete tumor removal.

- **Clinical features.** Spinal neuroblastomas are extradural in location and dumbbell shaped. They are located on the lower spinal cord from the mid-thoracic to the lumbosacral region. Partial or complete paralysis of both legs is present at birth. Urinary incontinence is more common than urinary retention. A palpable abdominal mass sometimes suggests the diagnosis.
- **Diagnosis.** Neuroimaging reveals the tumor mass.
- **Management.** Laminectomy, with partial or complete excision of tumor, is the rule. The advantage of adding radiotherapy and/or chemotherapy is not established. All survivors have some degree of paraparesis.

Teratoma

Teratomas of the spinal cord are similar in morphology, but less common in frequency, than teratomas of the brain. The tumor site can be at any level of the spinal cord, but definite predilection for the sacrum exists. Paraplegia or quadriplegia may be present, depending on the tumor location. Incontinence of urine and feces is a constant feature of sacral tumors and may occur with tumors at higher segmental levels.

Sacrococcygeal teratoma may erode through the vertebrae and present on the back as a cystic mass, caudal to the sacrum, displacing the rectum anteriorly. Neuroimaging shows calcification within the mass. Surgical extirpation of the tumor may be life saving, but permanent neurological sequelae are to be expected.

Neurocutaneous Syndromes

Neurocutaneous syndromes (phakomatoses) are a group of genetic or congenital disorders in which abnormalities of the nervous system are associated with either cutaneous features, ocular features, or both. Because the cutaneous features produce a birthmark, the term phakomatoses, meaning *mother spot* applies to the group. The cerebral abnormality results from disturbances of cellular proliferation, migration, and differentiation. Only a small number of neurocutaneous syndromes have clinical features in the newborn. The discussion of incontinentia pigmenti is in Chapter 2. This section deals with three relatively common syndromes: neurofibromatosis, tuberous sclerosis, and the Sturge–Weber syndrome.

Neurofibromatosis

- **Pathophysiology.** Neurofibromatosis (NF) is actually two different genetic diseases. NF type 1 (NF1) is probably the most common single-gene disorder of the nervous system, affecting 1 in 4000 individuals. A mutation of the NF1 gene on chromosome 17q causes the disorder. Approximately 100 mutations of NF1 are identifiable in the gene. Neurofibromin, the NF1 gene product, is partially homologous to GTPase-activating protein. Inheritance of the disorder is autosomal dominant, but one-half of cases result from a spontaneous mutation (Friedman, 2004).
- **Clinical features.** Dermatological evidence of disease is present at birth in 40% of cases. Early expression of symptoms is generally associated with severe involvement and serious complications. The severity of the disease is greater in children born to affected mothers than in those born to affected fathers or in those with neither parent affected. Café-au-lait spots, caused by excess melanin in the basal layer of the epidermis, are the only feature in the newborn. They appear as light brown, freckle-like lesions, 1–3 mm in diameter, in the axillae or intertriginous regions. Intracranial, intraspinal, and peripheral nerve tumors, features of neurofibromatosis in childhood and adult life, are rarely symptomatic in the newborn. Disturbances of cortical neuronal migration, subcortical heterotopias and disordered cortical lamination, account for the psychomotor retardation and seizures that develop in 20% of patients. Hydrocephalus from aqueductal stenosis occurs in 16% of infants, but not in the newborn. However, megalencephaly, due

to abnormal neuronal migration, is sometimes present at birth and may be a recurrent feature in some families. Enlargement of limbs, tongue, and internal organs due to plexiform neurofibromata occurs as well.
- **Diagnosis.** The cutaneous features are diagnostic. DNA testing is available but rarely needed. A family history of the disease raises suspicion and alerts the clinician to inspect the skin for café-au-lait spots. Brain MRI in newborns with seizures and café-au-lait spots often reveals migrational errors.
- **Management.** Management is symptomatic.

Tuberous Sclerosis

- **Pathophysiology.** Tuberous sclerosis is a disturbance in the differentiation of all embryonic germ layers. Genetic transmitted is an autosomal dominant trait with variable penetrance (Northrup and Au, 2004). Two genes are responsible for the phenotype. One gene (TSC1) is located at chromosome 9q34, and the other (TSC2) at chromosome 16p13.3. TSC1 more likely accounts for familial cases than TSC2 and is a less severe phenotype.

  The characteristic cerebral lesion is the tuber, a pale white nodule that grows in the cortex and in the ependymal lining. Subependymal *tubers*, consisting of glial cells and bizarre abnormal nerve cells project into the ventricle and produce a roughened surface. Tubers cause symptoms, not only because they are tumor masses, but also because they deprive the brain of its normal neuronal population. Neurons adjacent to cortical tubers are small, misshapen, and disoriented. Malignant transformation may occur in periventricular tubers but is uncommon in cortical tubers.
- **Clinical features.** The tissue dysplasis of tuberous sclerosis affect several organs. The only clinical features identifiable in the newborn are cardiorespiratory distress, due to rhabdomyoma of the heart, and depigmented areas of the skin. The depigmented areas measure 1 to 3 cm in diameter and are sharply demarcated from the normal skin. Tubers are present in the brain, even as early as 33 weeks' of gestation, but are asymptomatic.
- **Diagnosis.** An NIH consensus panel established criteria for the diagnosis of tuberous complex (Roach et al., 1999). However, these criteria have limited use in the newborn. Because the clinical expression of the trait is variable, it is difficult to predict the outcome for a newborn with tuberous sclerosis. Molecular diagnosis is available for both types but mainly used for diagnostic confirmation or prenatal testing. Neurological dysfunction, when present, generally becomes apparent during infancy.
- **Management.** Newborns rarely require intervention, but follow-up screening for cerebral, renal, and cardiac tumors is the rule.

Sturge–Weber syndrome

- **Pathophysiology.** Sturge–Weber syndrome has no established genetic basis. The complete syndrome consists of a port wine stain (angioma) on the upper part of the face, ipsilateral leptomeningeal telangiectasia, contralateral seizures and hemiparesis, and mental retardation. The vascular abnormalities are persistent primitive blood vessels that appear in early fetal life over the brain and face and undergo complete involution. The facial angioma consists of endothelial lined vessels surrounded by a thin layer of collagen. The blood is venous, under low pressure, with no clear-cut direction of flow. The intracranial telangiectasia is in the pia, usually over the parieto-occipital region of one hemisphere, and does not invade the cortex. A colloid protein with an affinity to bind calcium salts transudes through the abnormal vessels into the meninges and subjacent layers of cortex. Cortical neurons are lost and calcification develops in the gyri.

- **Clinical features.** The facial angioma is present at birth and often has a sharp, midline demarcation in the area supplied by the ophthalmic division of the trigeminal nerve. This localization is so constant that the minimal lesion is an angioma above the lateral angle of the eye. Angiomas sometimes cross the midline or extend to the lips, neck, and chest. Involvement of deeper tissues causes hypertrophy of the eyelids, the lips, or both. Seizures occur in 90% of children and have their onset in the first weeks or months.

  Occasional children have the characteristic neurological and neuroimaging features without skin lesion. More frequently, the typical cutaneous and ophthalmic findings are unassociated with clinical or neuroimaging evidence of intracranial lesions. Although the leptomeningeal angioma is typically ipsilateral to a unilateral facial nevus, bilateral brain lesions occur in at least 15% of children.

- **Diagnosis.** The combination of the facial angioma and seizures are diagnostic. MRI with gadolinium contrast demonstrates the abnormal intracranial vessels. The leptomeningeal angioma is typically ipsilateral to the facial nevus. Bilateral brain lesions occur in at least 15% of patients.

- **Management.** Hemispherectomy is the recommended treatment for newborns with intractable seizures. The procedure improves seizure control and promotes better intellectual development (Kossoff et al., 2002).

REFERENCES

Dodge NN and Dobyns WB. Agenesis of the corpus callosum and Dandy–Walker malformation associated with hemimeganencephaly in the sebaceous nevus syndrome. Am J Med Genet 1995;56:147–150.

Fort DW and Rushing EJ. Congenital central nervous system tumors. J Child Neurol 1997;12:157–164.

Friedman JM. Neurofibromatosis 1. (Updated 5 October, 2004). In: GeneClinics: Medical Genetics Knowledge Base [database online]. University of Washington at Seattle. Available at http://www.geneclinics.org

Haverkamp F, Wolfle J, Aretz M, et al. Congenital hydrocephalus internus and aqueduct stenosis: aetiology and implications for genetic counselling. Eur J Pediat 1999;158:474–478.

Kossoff EH, Buck C, Freeman JM. Outcomes of 32 hemispherectomies for Sturge–Weber syndrome worldwide. Neurology 2002;59:1735–1738.

Northrup H and Au K-S. Tuberous sclerosis complex. (Updated 27 September 2004) In: GeneClinics: Medical Genetics Knowledge Base [database online]. University of Washington at Seattle. Available at http://www.geneclinics.org

Harper PS and Upadhyaya M. Molecular genetics of neurofibromatosis type 1 (NF1). J Med Genet 1996;33:2–17.

Roach ES, Gomez MR and Northrup H. Tuberous sclerosis complex consensus conference: revised clinical diagnostic criteria. J Child Neurol 1999;13:624–628.

Schrander-Stumpel C and Vos YJ. L1 syndrome. (Updated 29 April 2004) In: GeneClinics: Medical Genetics Knowledge Base [database online]. University of Washington at Seattle. Available at http://www.geneclinics.org

Wakeling EL, Jolly M, Fisk NM, et al. X-linked inheritance of Dandy–Walker variant. Clin Dysmorph 2002;11:15–18.

10

Electroencephalography and Evoked Response

Gregory N. Barnes

This text stresses the importance of magnetic resonance imaging (MRI), computed tomography (CT) and ultrasound (US) in refining neurological diagnosis in the newborn. However, imaging modalities have limited usefulness in defining normal and abnormal brain physiological function. Electroencephalography (EEG) and evoked response (EVR) complement MRI, CT, and US by defining normal and abnormal electrical activity of cortical and subcortical brain regions. These laboratory studies add immeasurably to, but do not replace, the information derived from attentive history-taking, careful examination, and continuous concern (see Ch. 1).

EEG METHODOLOGY

The expertise and the interest of the technician performing the studies are critical factors to the success of the laboratory. Special training is required, mostly acquired through experience, in the techniques of neonatal EEG and in the procedures of an intensive care nursery. Clinical observations of the newborn by the technician are crucial to the success of the enterprise. Very sick newborns in an intensive care unit are the setting for most studies. The equipment attached to and surrounding the newborn (used for monitoring and supporting vital function) is not only a physical obstacle but also a potential source of considerable electrical interference. It is the technician's responsibility to designate artifacts, categorize states of sleep and wakefulness, and record subtle alterations in the posture and movement of the child.

A 21-channel EEG machine is optimal for neonatal studies; 16 channels monitor EEG and five monitor noncerebral functions. The noncerebral channels are one for electrocardiogram (EKG), one for electromyogram (EMG), two for electro-oculogram (EOG), and one for respiratory monitoring. However, in many newborns, 10 channels of EEG are adequate.

199

In addition to standard EEG studies, Video EEG (V/EEG) system is useful for prolonged EEG monitoring (24 to 48 hours). The V/EEG records digitally all 21 channels of data and stores the information on a compact disc (CD). Twenty-four hours of data may be stored on one CD and then displayed for analysis on a computer workstation.

Placement of Electrodes

- **EEG.** Silver cup electrodes are applied using electrode paste and gauze squares. Electrode impedances are under 10,000 ohms but more than 100 ohms. The International Ten Twenty Electrode Placement System is the standard used to measure the head for electrode placement. Mastoid leads substitute for A1 and A2.
- **EKG.** Two silver cup electrodes, filled with electrode paste, are used. One taped to the right arm and one to the left leg. The two electrodes reference to each other.
- **EMG.** Two silver cup electrodes, filled with electrode paste, are used. One is taped 0.5 cm above the outer canthus of the right eye, and the other is taped 0.5 cm below the outer canthus of the left eye. Each references individually to the A1 electrode on the left mastoid. This electrode arrangement produces an out-of-phase deflection for eye movements.
- **Respiration.** In newborns not intubated, a thermocouple recorder, taped to the nose, provides an excellent display of the respiratory pattern. Premature and term newborns require different sizes of thermocouples. In intubated newborns, a piezoelectric transducer taped to the right side of the abdomen substitutes for the thermocouple recorder. However, recordings obtained from the piezoelectric transducer are more easily distorted by extraneous movements of the child and technically inferior to those obtained by the thermocouple. A standard EEG channel records respirations.
- **V/EEG.** Scalp electrode placement, secured with paste, are at the F1, F2, T3, T4, C3, C4, 01, and 02 positions when using all four channels for EEG recording. When an EKG is required as well, place adjacent electrodes at the F7 or F8 position and at the T5 or T6 position.

Instrumentation and Recording

EEG montages vary from laboratory to laboratory and generally designed to meet the personal preference of the electroencephalographer or the requirements of a research study design. For standard EEG, use a single montage throughout the recording. The standard longitudinal bipolar montage records 16 channels of EEG. Because the first five channels are noncerebral leads, the EEG channels are designated 6 to 15. Scalp-to-scalp montages are the routine for recording. Montages using referential electrodes, other than an average reference, are of limited usefulness because of the distortion of EKG (and other) artifacts.

Table 10–1 summarizes the sensitivity and filters used for each of the recording function in standard neonatal EEG. Paper speed is 30 mm/sec; and further slowed to 15 mm/sec when asymmetries appear that require further evaluation. A 60-minute recording is required to examine fully the wakefulness and sleep cycles of the neonate. Prolonged V/EEG recordings are preferable in sick newborns with decreased states of consciousness and continued electrical or clinical seizures despite maximal treatments. Nursery staff who must attend to the child's health needs frequently interrupt studies on sick newborns. Test the reactivity of EEG patterns during normal states (sleep) and abnormal states (decreased consciousness, seizures) with photic, auditory, and/or tactile stimulation.

NORMAL EEG PATTERNS

Defining Wakefulness and Sleep States

The technician judge's wakefulness based on behavioral observations (eyes open, crying, body movements) rather than by the use of electrophysiological monitoring (Anders et al., 1971). The recognition of sleep onset is by behavioral observations as well, but the definition of sleep states requires a combination of observational and monitoring criteria. The three sleep states recognized in the newborn: active sleep, quiet sleep, and indeterminate or transitional sleep. Table 10–2 summarizes the monitoring criteria for each state.

TABLE 10–1   Sensitivity and filters

Monitor	Sensitivity (uV/mm)	High freq filter (c/sec)	Low freq filter (c/sec)
EKG	70	15	1
EMG	5	70	5
EOG	7	35	3
Respiration	Variable	15	1
EEG	7 varied during the recording	70	1 varied during the recording

TABLE 10–2   Determination of sleep states

Sleep state	EMG	EOG	EEG	Respiration
Active	Movements present	Movements present	Continuous	Irregular
Quiet	Movements absent	Movements absent	Discontinuous	Regular
Indeterminate	Movements absent	Movements absent	Sleep intervals that do not meet the criteria for active or quiet sleep	

Active Sleep

Active sleep, the equivalent of rapid eye movement (REM) sleep, is the predominant sleep pattern of the premature, and it occupies approximately 50% of sleep time at term (Parmelee et al., 1968). Newborns rarely enter active sleep directly from wakefulness. The EOG records continuous or intermittent eye movements and one observes intermittent migratory movements in the face and limbs, sometimes associated with smiling, grimacing, or crying. The EMG records these random movements, which vary in duration, frequency, and amplitude. Respiration is irregular, often with episodes of apnea. Heart rate is regular, but may become irregular with the apnea.

Quiet Sleep

Quiet sleep occupies less than 20% of total sleep time at 30 weeks' gestation, 40% at term, and more than 50% during infancy. No recorded eye movements or observed face and limbs occur. EMG demonstrates continuous low-level activity. Respiration and heart rate are regular.

Indeterminate Sleep

Epochs of monitoring that do not fit the criteria for active or quiet sleep are termed indeterminate. Such epochs occur most often at sleep onset, when sleep states are changing, and in premature newborns.

EEG Ontogenesis

Normal patterns of EEG activity have been established for human premature newborns of 25 weeks conceptional age and older. The rich variety of patterns observed is difficult to categorize completely, but a predictable maturational sequence has been constructed (Watanabe et al., 1980; Werner et al., 1977). Important trends in EEG ontogenesis include the development of a continuous background, the progressive differentiation of sleep states, a reduction in the number of normal spikes and sharp waves, the development of occipital predominance, and an increased reactivity to stimuli.

The major focus of a clinical EEG laboratory is to identify abnormal cerebral states. For this purpose, it is convenient to divide the normal EEG into four conceptional age-related patterns: 25 to 31 weeks, 32 to 34 weeks, 35 to 37 weeks, and 38 to 42 weeks. This age division, like any age division, is arbitrary; the ontogenesis of the brain and its electrical rhythms are a continuous process.

25 to 31 Weeks

Active sleep occupies more than 70% of total sleep time (Fig. 10–1). Monitoring criteria cannot differentiate active sleep and wakefulness and the determination

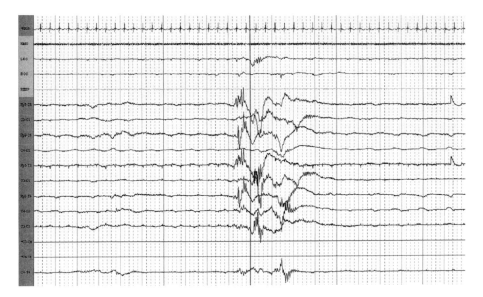

FIGURE 10–1   Active sleep, 25 to 31 weeks. The record is almost continuous and consists of slow waves with superimposed faster frequencies. (Courtesy of Dr Bassel Abou-Khalil, Professor of Neurology, Vanderbilt University School of Medicine and Director of The Vanderbilt Epilepsy Division and Clinical Neurophysiology Training Program, Vanderbilt Medical Center.)

is by behavioral observations. Differentiating active sleep and quiet sleep is mainly by noncerebral monitors, especially before 30 weeks. The characteristic feature of the EEG, discontinuity of the record, is more prominent in quiet sleep than active sleep. Intervals of background suppression are interrupted by bursts of high-amplitude (100 to 300 μV) slow waves with superimposed sharp waves and spikes. The average duration of complete suppression is 4 seconds at 27 weeks and 2 seconds at term. The longest duration of complete suppression is 14 seconds at 27 weeks and 3 seconds at term (Hahn et al., 1989). Burst duration is 3 to 10 seconds at 27 weeks and three to six seconds at 31 weeks. The longest acceptable inter-burst intervals are 27–46 seconds in 26–28 weeks (Selton et al., 2000) and 20–35 seconds in 29–33 weeks (Hahn et al., 1989; Clancy et al., 2003).

Rhythmic activity in all frequencies is abundant. Delta is more prominent from the occipital region, and alpha and beta from the central region. Three delineated recognizable patterns of activity are delta brushes, sawtooths, and frontal transients. Delta brushes consist of a slow wave (0.5 to 1.5 c/sec, 70 to 250 μV) with superimposed rhythmic activity (8 to 22 c/sec, 30 to 225 μV) (Fig. 10–1). Their distribution is diffuse at first, but then develops a central and occipital predominance until they disappear at 36–37 weeks. Delta brushes occur with greatest frequency at 30 to 31 weeks when they are most abundant during active sleep.

Sawtooths (also called temporal theta or temporal alpha) are bursts of sharp rhythmic 4 to 7 c/sec waves with amplitudes of 100 to 250 μV that appear in the temporal region by 26 weeks and disappear by 32–34 weeks. Spikes and sharp transients are a constant feature in the EEGs of normal premature and term newborns (Fig. 10–2). At 31 weeks, they appear in all locations, synchronously or nonsynchronously between the two hemispheres (Veechierini-Blineau et al., 1996). Frontal sharp transients refer to biphasic waves that may be isolated or repetitive at a frequency of 1 c/sec.

Normal spike and sharp wave transients may be difficult to distinguish from abnormal electroconvulsive discharges. The criteria that help identify electro-convulsive discharges, but are not absolute, are repetition, rhythmicity, amplitude, symmetry, and persistent focality. In general, rare temporal sharp waves with voltage <75 μV and duration <100 ms are normal. Conversely, frequent focal temporal sharp waves that exceed 150 μV in amplitude and are greater than 150 ms in duration are likely abnormal (Mizrahi et al., 2003). Likewise, a temporal sharp wave in the EEG record of an awake term infant is also abnormal.

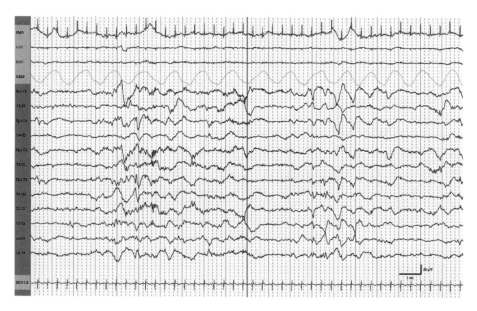

FIGURE 10–2   Twenty-second page demonstrating 'tracé alternant' pattern, a normal pattern of quiet sleep (equivalent to slow wave sleep in adults). There are 4–6 second periods of higher voltage activity alternating with 4–6 seconds of lower voltage. This is not burst suppression because the lower voltage periods still have EEG activity, and because this pattern will be reactive when the patient is stimulated. (Courtesy of Dr Bassel Abou-Khalil, Professor of Neurology, Vanderbilt University School of Medicine and Director of The Vanderbilt Epilepsy Division and Clinical Neurophysiology Training Program, Vanderbilt Medical Center.)

32 to 34 Weeks

At this age, the EEG patterns of active sleep and quiet sleep differentiate, but active sleep and wakefulness are only distinguishable by behavioral observation. A characteristic feature of the EEG at 32 to 34 weeks is an increase in the frequency of spike and sharp wave transients. Their appearance is random and multifocal in distribution.

Active Sleep and Wakefulness The background is more continuous, but still demonstrates some episodes of discontinuity. Occipital-predominant slow wave activity develops at 30 weeks and well established by 32 weeks. The spindle component of delta brushes, without a well-developed slow wave component, may appear in the central and occipital regions.

Quiet Sleep The record remains discontinuous, but the periods of discontinuity are shorter in duration and contain low-amplitude fast frequencies. Recorded during the bursts of activity are delta brushes, occipital slow waves, and central spikes. Rhythmic 1.5 Hz activity appears in the frontal regions. Temporal alpha bursts replace temporal theta at 33 weeks and disappear by 35 weeks. Interval burst intervals do not exceed 10–20 seconds (Hahn et al., 1989; Clancy et al., 2003).

35 to 37 Weeks

Active sleep and quiet sleep are easily differentiated by both behavioral and EEG characteristics. Diffuse attenuation occurs in all states as a response to stimulation. Spike and sharp wave transients decrease in frequency and occur mainly during the burst phase of quiet sleep.

Active Sleep and Wakefulness The background is continuous and consists of low-amplitude (5 to 30 µV) fast frequencies and higher-amplitude (20 to 100 µV) theta and delta. Beta activity has an anterior predominance, and delta activity has a posterior predominance. Delta brushes are no longer present.

Quiet Sleep The record remains discontinuous, but is undergoing evolution into the pattern of trace alternant characteristic mature newborn EEG. Sharp transients tend to occur only during the burst phase, with the exception of high-amplitude frontal sharp waves. Interhemispheric synchrony of the bursts increases from 60% to 80% to 90%. The longest acceptable interburst interval is 5–10 seconds (Clancy et al., 2003).

38 to 42 Weeks

The EEG is continuous, and all states of sleep and wakefulness are distinguishable. Behavioral observations are still important in distinguishing active sleep from wakefulness because the EEG patterns are similar. Occipital predominance is declining, and slow wave activity distributes diffusely over the hemispheres (Joseph et al., 1976). Immature waveforms decrease in frequency: (1) Delta brushes are uncommon and being replaced by rhythmic beta; (2) Spike and sharp wave transients are more sporadic, multifocal in distribution, and are recorded mainly during quiet sleep in the burst phase of the trace alternant pattern (Statz et al., 1982); (3) Frontal sharp transients are still frequent, generally bilateral, but sometimes unilateral, and present during wakefulness and quiet sleep. All of these patterns will decrease in frequency in the ensuing weeks.

Wakefulness   The background is continuous and consists, for the most part, of low-amplitude (5 to 30 μV) 5 to 7 c/sec waves distributed uniformly over the hemispheres (Fig. 10–3). Sharp transients are common from the frontal electrodes, but uncommon in other locations. Muscle artifact caused by crying, sucking, and limb movement frequently interrupted the background. Sharp transients tend to resolve by 44–48 weeks and temporal sharp waves in a waking EEG at term are abnormal (Mizrahi et al., 2003).

Active Sleep   Active sleep occupies 50% of total sleep time. The background is continuous and contains mixed frequencies (5 to 12 c/sec) of low amplitude distributed uniformly over the hemispheres (Fig. 10–4). Fifty percent of newborns show rhythmic activity, 7 to 10 c/sec and 20 to 30 μV, in the frontal and

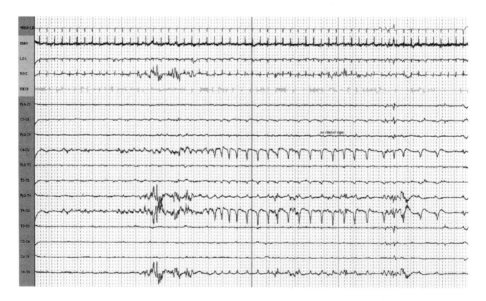

FIGURE 10–3   Right occipital ictal discharge displayed on a 30-second page. (Courtesy of Dr Bassel Abou-Khalil, Professor of Neurology, Vanderbilt University School of Medicine and Director of The Vanderbilt Epilepsy Division and Clinical Neurophysiology Training Program, Vanderbilt Medical Center.)

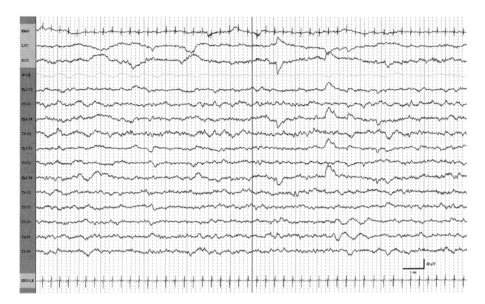

FIGURE 10–4 Twenty-second page demonstrating activité moyenne in active sleep in a 27-day term infant; note rapid eye movements, absence of muscle artifact, and irregular respiration. (Courtesy of Dr Bassel Abou-Khalil, Professor of Neurology, Vanderbilt University School of Medicine and Director of The Vanderbilt Epilepsy Division and Clinical Neurophysiology Training Program, Vanderbilt Medical Center.)

central regions (Statz et al., 1982). Slow waves may be intermixed in the background but are not a dominant rhythm.

Quiet Sleep Two patterns of quiet sleep exist. One consists of diffuse and continuous slow wave activity (Fig. 10–1) and the other is a bursting pattern, termed the *trace alternant* (Fig. 10–2). The term trace alternant is different from the discontinuous pattern of the premature and correctly used only in reference to the term newborn in quiet sleep. Bursts of slow wave (1 to 3 c/sec) of 50 to 100 μV appear every 4 to 5 seconds which may be intermixed with a spindling beta (14 to 20 c/sec). Activity is present also between bursts; it consists of faster frequencies (4 to 7 c/sec) of low amplitude (50 μV). The trace alternant pattern resolves by 44 weeks.

ABNORMAL EEG PATTERNS

Neonatal EEG has its greatest value in determining the severity of an acute encephalopathy secondary to perinatal asphyxia and in determining whether seizure activity is present. Hypoxic-ischemic encephalopathy provides the most accurate correlation between the cerebral and the EEG states. The correlation is sufficiently high that a marked discrepancy between the state of consciousness and the severity of the EEG disturbance should suggest an etiology other than hypoxic-ischemic encephalopathy.

It is useful to divide abnormal EEG patterns as mild and severe. Mild abnormalities are those in which the outcome for eventual neurological outcome is not certain; severe abnormalities are usually associated with an unfavorable outcome.

Mild EEG Abnormalities

Background disorganization or immaturity, in the absence of marked amplitude suppression or an electroconvulsive discharge, is a common feature of mild EEG abnormalities. Transitory mild abnormalities are unlikely to be significant.

Lack of Variability

The most common mild EEG abnormality is a background of continuous, mostly slow, mixed frequencies of normal amplitude that does not vary with sleep states or external stimulation. Because not all states of sleep and wakefulness are fully distinguishable in normal newborns of less than 37 to 38 weeks' conceptional age, lack of variability is more characteristic at term than in prematures.

In prematures of 30 weeks' gestation or greater, lack of variability may be recognized as either generalized low-voltage with normal background or as poorly developed occipital delta. Approximately one-third of such prematures will be normal, somewhat more than one-third will survive with a neurological handicap, and the remainder die (Tharp et al., 1981). Death among prematures is more often from cardiorespiratory than from cerebral causes. Do not presume that prematures who die would have had an unfavorable neurological outcome if they had survived. In preterm infants with cerebral hemorrhage, the degree of background depression correlates with the extent of brain damage and with the grade of IVH (Clancy et al., 1984; Benda et al., 1989; Aso et al., 1993). Mild prolonged depression in early life EEGs of preterm infants followed by EEG dysmaturity at 40 weeks is associated with later cognitive impairment (Ferrari et al., 1992; Biagnoni et al., 1996).

Asymmetries

Most asymmetries of amplitude and frequency in the background rhythms are positional and readily corrected by straightening the head. Asymmetries that are not positional in origin are not necessarily significant. Transitory amplitude asymmetries are common in 3–4% of all newborns (O'Brien et al., 1987), tend to vary in location, and considered normal unless there is also background suppression. Persistent amplitude asymmetries of 50% or greater between hemispheres, especially when associated with a frequency asymmetry, may indicate a structural abnormality in the hemisphere with amplitude attenuation. Infarction or intracerebral hemorrhage is often the cause in term newborn (Fenichel et al.,

1983). Focal slow wave activity may be present in a destructive lesion. In term infants, these focal slow waves may indicate congenital anomalies of the brain. In the premature, persistent amplitude asymmetries correlate with bad neurological outcomes or death, and may indicate the side of periventricular hemorrhagic infarction (Aso et al., 1989).

Positive Rolandic Sharp Waves

Positive Rolandic sharp waves (PRSW) with a steep initial positive slope localized to the central electrodes were described in prematures with intraventricular hemorrhage before the use of routine ultrasound examinations (see Ch. 4). Once thought an important indicator of intracranial hemorrhage, they correlate better with gestational age than with hemorrhage (Clancy and Tharp, 1984; Lacey et al., 1986). These waves are not specific for IVH but indicate white matter necrosis. Studies by Marret et al. (1992) of 300 preterm infants indicate that the absence of PRSW in neonatal EEGs correlates with a favorable motor outcome in 98%. The presence of two or more PRSW per minute correlates well with the development of spastic diplegia. PRSW are early markers of white matter damage. PRSW appear in the first week after birth and may precede the development of cysts characteristic of PVL on cranial ultrasound (Baud et al., 1998). PRSW can also be seen in meningitis, hydrocephalus, aminoacidurias (Tharp et al., 1981) and HIE (Mizrahi et al., 2003). The rate of recurrence of PRSW in excess of two waves per second is associated with a poor developmental outcome (Blume and Dreyfus-Brisac, 1982).

Focal temporal and extratemporal sharp waves or spikes may occur in the frontal, temporal, central, or occipital regions. When the waves or spikes have sufficient amplitude, duration, polarity, and are persistently focal, their presence indicates a focal brain injury. The persistence of temporal sharp waves in neonatal EEGs could indicate a child at risk for postneonatal epilepsy, especially if there is a family history of epilepsy (Clancy and Legido, 1991; Barnes et al., 2006). Multiple sharp wave foci of high-voltage and long duration indicate a diffuse CNS injury. The multifocal sharp waves are predominant over the temporal regions and may be more prominent over one hemisphere. The significance of multiple focal sharp waves for prediction of epileptogenicity and long-term neurodevelopmental outcome is unclear.

Record Immaturity

Some recorded EEG patterns seem immature for the conceptional age as determined by other parameters of maturity. In such newborns, the history or physical examination often suggests the occurrence of cerebral stress. In some newborns, the clinical history and neurological examination complement the immature EEG record, suggesting delayed myelination and a possible intrauterine cerebral insult. However, since most requests for EEGs are because of suspected abnormal neurological function, the significance of the association between record immaturity and cerebral stress is uncertain.

A single immature EEG in a premature newborn (immature defined as discrepant by at least 2 weeks) does not indicate an unfavorable outcome (Tharp et al., 1981). However, serial EEGs that demonstrate a persistent immaturity over several weeks or a regression from normal maturity to immaturity are associated with an increased incidence of chronic neurological handicap (Lombroso, 1982).

Sleep Cycle Modifications

Several investigators have indicated that certain specific disorders, especially hypoxia, may lengthen or shorten the relative duration of active or quiet sleep (Holmes et al., 1979; Watanabe et al., 1980). The actual number of studies in hypoxic-ischemic infants is few (Garcias Da Silva et al., 2004; Osredkar et al., 2005). For most disorders, the degree of sleep cycle modification, in relationship to normal variability, is not impressive (3–5% of all infants). Further, the relative percentage of quiet and active sleep is sufficiently variable from newborn-to-newborn that a single recording in the first postnatal week is not conclusive.

Severe EEG Abnormalities

Suppression of the background and electroconvulsive discharges always indicates a marked disturbance in cerebral function and an unfavorable outcome.

Suppression of the Background

Electrocerebral Silence   The EEG definition of electrocerebral silence used for older children and adults (no electrical activity over $2\mu V$ between scalp or referential electrode pairs 10 or more cm apart, with electrode impedances under 10,000 ohms but more than 100 ohms) is applicable to the newborn as well. However, the recording of electrocerebral silence does not equate with brain death in the fetus and newborn. During labor, transitory periods of electrocerebral silence occur in the fetus. These periods correlate well with the severity of fetal acidosis (Wilson et al., 1979). An inactive EEG also occurs in prematures with hypothermia and in newborns of all ages exposed to high doses of maternal anesthesia and analgesia (Tharp et al., 1981). Persistent electrocerebral silence is associated with widespread encephalomalacia of grey matter (Aso et al., 1989) or hydranencephaly and portends an unfavorable outcome. Prolonged survival occurs in infants with electrocerebral silence (Mizrahi et al., 1985).

Decreased Voltage   Recordings with amplitudes that are constantly less than ten to $15\mu V$, especially when lacking frequency variability (Fig. l0–5) are always indicative of severe brain damage with subsequent neurological abnormalities in survivors (Lombroso and Holmes, 1993). Progressive decline in amplitude is a particularly grave sign and may end in electrocerebral silence.

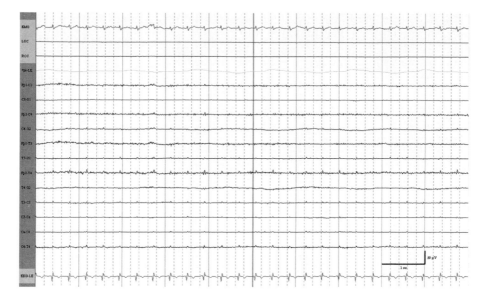

FIGURE 10–5 Generalized attenuation in a 3-day-old with hypoxic ischemic encephalopathy. (Courtesy of Dr Bassel Abou-Khalil, Professor of Neurology, Vanderbilt University School of Medicine and Director of The Vanderbilt Epilepsy Division and Clinical Neurophysiology Training Program, Vanderbilt Medical Center.)

Attenuation of the background is a particularly sensitive index of the severity, and therefore the outcome, of HIE (Holmes et al., 1982; Watanabe et al., 1980). In a term newborn experiencing seizures, if the EEG has a normal background, consider an etiology other than HIE. Background attenuation occurs in severe metabolic disorders, meningitis/encephalitis, cerebral hemorrhage, and IVH.

Burst Suppression   In prematures of 25 to 31 weeks, the normal background has a burst suppression appearance. This appearance continues, with modification, after 31 weeks during quiet sleep. Burst suppression is not pathological in prematures younger than 34 weeks. Burst suppression in term newborns is characterized by intervals of suppression (less than 5 μV) interrupted by bursts of disorganized activity (Fig. 10–6). This pattern is always associated with an unfavorable outcome and correlates with severe neuronal necrosis (Grigg-Damberger et al., 1989; Clancy and Legido, 1991; Ortibus et al., 1996). Burst suppression is also associated with the development of post-neonatal epilepsy, especially if the EEG is nonreactive (Clancy and Legido, 1991; Nunes et al., 2005; Barnes et al., 2006).

Burst suppression occurs most often in newborns with severe HIE and in metabolic disorders. It is a common feature in the EEG of newborns with glycine encephalopathy (see Ch. 7). In such newborns, the burst suppression pattern evolves into hypsarrhythmia with time (Markand et al., 1982).

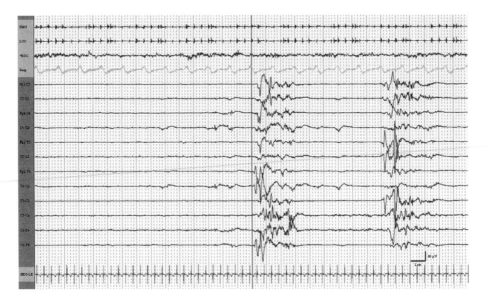

FIGURE 10–6 Burst suppression pattern: 1-day-old premature (33-week gestation) with multiple congenital anomalies. (Courtesy of Dr Bassel Abou-Khalil, Professor of Neurology, Vanderbilt University School of Medicine and Director of The Vanderbilt Epilepsy Division and Clinical Neurophysiology Training Program, Vanderbilt Medical Center.)

Electroconvulsive Discharges

Although rare before 34–35 weeks CA, electroconvulsive discharges are both repetitive and rhythmic. With increasing conceptual age, electrical seizures become longer in duration and more frequent on neonatal EEG (Scher et al., 1993). Rhythmicity is the feature that most clearly distinguishes electroconvulsive discharges from normal sharp transients. Most electroconvulsive discharges are focal in onset; some remain focal and others become generalized. The initial focus may shift or remain constant during a single recording. Most electrical seizures arise from the temporal or central regions (Patrizi et al., 2003) (Fig. 10–7). A constant focus may indicate a focal brain disturbance, especially cerebral infarction or hemorrhage in the term newborn (Fenichel et al., 1983).

However, generalized or regional onset of ictal discharges may follow either a focal or generalized brain disturbance in preterm and term infants. Interestingly, full term infants have sharp waves, spikes, sharp and slow waves, and spike and slow waves at ictal onset whereas in preterm infants rhythmic delta activity was more common. No consistent relationship exists between etiology and the onset, morphology, frequency, or propagation of ictal patterns in either term or preterm infants. In general, clinical seizure activity occurs more commonly with electrographic seizures when the EEG background is normal or mild to moderately abnormal than when the background is severely abnormal (Patrizi et al., 2003).

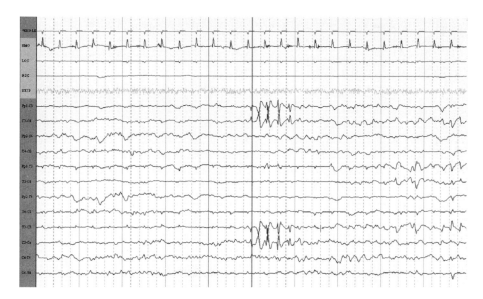

FIGURE 10–7 Abnormal train of sharp waves at C3. (Courtesy of Dr Bassel Abou-Khalil, Professor of Neurology, Vanderbilt University School of Medicine and Director of The Vanderbilt Epilepsy Division and Clinical Neurophysiology Training Program, Vanderbilt Medical Center.)

Continuous EEG monitoring is the only method to detect seizures in newborns paralyzed with muscle relaxants to aid respiratory assistance (see Ch. 2). Monitoring is useful as well to identify newborns having electroconvulsive discharges in the absence of clinical manifestations. The variety of patterns recognizable as electroconvulsive discharges is considerable. It is convenient to divide these patterns into three groups: slow (flat) spike discharges, monorhythmic discharges, and repetitive single spike discharges.

Slow (Flat) Spike Discharges Slow spike discharges, a common form of electroconvulsive discharge in the newborn, are characterized by repetitive slow waves (approximately 1 c/sec) of 50 μV or less which usually demonstrate a phase reversal at a single electrode. The discharge may remain localized, spread to adjacent electrodes in the same hemisphere, or shift to the opposite hemisphere.

Monorhythmic Discharges These discharges begin as repetitive waves of a single frequency and need not be sharp waves (Fig. 10–3). The frequency of the discharge may shift during the seizure, but the focus usually remains constant (Fig. 10–7). Alpha (8 to 15 c/sec) discharges are generally of lower amplitude than theta (4 to 7 c/sec) discharges or delta (1 to 3 c/sec) discharges. Phase reversals may or may not be present. The duration of discharge is variable but tends to be longer in duration. Monorhythmic alpha discharges generally localize to the Rolandic area (Knauss and Carlson, 1978). Prolonged monorhythmic discharges usually occur in newborns with states of decreased consciousness. The EEG background is usually depressed and undifferentiated. Brief monorhythmic discharges often occur without clinical manifestations. The presence of this pattern suggests a poor prognosis.

Repetitive Single Spike Discharges   Repetitive single spike discharges are relatively common in newborns with states of decreased consciousness. Intervals of background suppression separate single, well-defined spikes. At times, the spikes may have a periodic pattern. Periodic lateralizing epileptiform discharges (PLEDS) indicate an unfavorable outcome. PLEDS occur in asphyxiated newborns, those with herpes simplex encephalitis (McCutchen et al., 1985), and in other CNS disorders including cerebral infarction (Scher and Beggarly, 1989).

EVOKED RESPONSES

Sensory stimulation evokes an electrical potential in the brain in response to the stimulus. With the exception of the potentials evoked in the occipital cortex by flashing lights in the eyes, the evoked potentials of other sensory systems are too small to differentiate from the EEG background. Even the visual evoked response is not regularly distinguishable.

Commercially available instruments allow the detection of evoked responses following stimulation of the auditory, visual, and somatosensory systems. The basic principal is the same for all three modalities. A computer program detects the electrical potential in the brain time-locked to a sensory stimuli presented at a regular repetitive rate. The number of repetitions needed is inversely proportional to the amplitude of the evoked response. Evoked response testing provides information on the latency of sensory conduction in the central nervous system, the required time for information to travel from one point to another. In the newborn, this information is useful in assessing the maturation of the nervous system and the anatomical integrity of the sensory pathways.

Brainstem Auditory Evoked Response (BAER)

Methods

In measuring the brainstem auditory evoked response (BAER), electrodes are fixed to the vertex (Cz), forehead (Fz), and both mastoids using electrode paste and gauze squares. The vertex electrode is active, the mastoid electrodes are referential, and the forehead electrode is ground. This montage displays positive waves as an upward deflection. Each ear is stimulated at sound pressure levels about 70 decibels (dB), sufficient to produce a response. The stimulus is 2000 clicks presented at a rate of 10 per second, produced by an $100 \mu s$ square wave in the rarefaction acoustic phase. While stimulating one ear, the other hears white noise.

Evoked potentials record between the forehead and the ipsilateral mastoid and between the forehead and the contralateral mastoid. In the normal newborn, roman numerals number the five waves recorded from the forehead and the ipsi-lateral mastoid derivation. Wave I is generated by the acoustic nerve; wave II by the cochlear nuclei; wave III by the superior olivary complex; wave IV by the lateral lemniscus; and wave V by the inferior colliculus. Waves IV and V may be joined as a single or bifid wave. The simultaneously recorded forehead to contra-lateral mastoid derivations helps identify waves: wave I is absent, wave II holds its position, wave III attenuates, and waves IV and V separate. Several investigators established normal values for the absolute latency of waves I and V, the relative amplitudes of waves I and V, and the I to V interpeak interval. Table 10–3 sum-marizes the values of Despland and Galambos (1980). However, each laboratory must establish normal values for its own equipment and environment.

Maturation of the BAER

The ipsilaterally recorded BAER first appears at a conceptional age of 26 to 27 weeks in response to a stimulus intensity 60 to 70 dB above the hearing thresh-old of normal adults; the contralaterally recorded BAER appears after 31 weeks (Salamy et al., 1985). The absolute latencies of waves I and V and the V-I inter-peak interval decline progressively with advancing conceptional age (Vles et al., 1987). A later study using magnetoencephalography (MEG) in human fetuses and newborns reached a similar conclusion (Holst et al., 2005). The latencies of waves I and V, especially V, bear an inverse relationship to the intensity of the stimulus (Table 10–3).

The V-1 interpeak interval represents the time required for central conduction in the auditory system. There is general agreement that at 40 weeks concep-tional age the V-I interpeak interval is approximately 5.1 ms when the ear is stimulated at an intensity of 55 to 65 dB above adult hearing threshold. At 26 weeks' conceptional age, the V-I interpeak interval is 9.9 ms. The rapid decline in brainstem conduction time, attributed to myelination, is assessable in relation to the presence or absence of apnea in prematures. The V-1 interpeak interval is longer in prematures with apnea as compared with those without apnea at a similar conceptional age (Henderson-Smart et al., 1983). In prematures from 30 to 37 weeks' conceptional age, those without apnea have a V-1 interpeak interval of 5.68 ms or less at a stimulus intensity of 70 dB above adult threshold;

TABLE 10–3 Baer latencies (ms)[*]

Conceptional age	Wave I	Wave V	V-1 interval
30–31 weeks	Mean 3.50+3SD 5.09	Mean 9.10+3SD 10.06	Mean 5.60+3SD 7.25
32–33 weeks	Mean 2.78+3SD 3.44	Mean 8.36+3SD 9.98	Mean 5.62+3SD 6.52
34–35 weeks	Mean 2.56+3SD 3.31	Mean 8.00+3SD 9.41	Mean 5.44+3SD 6.41
36–37 weeks	Mean 2.53+3SD 3.10	Mean 7.80+3SD 9.42	Mean 5.27+3SD 6.42
38–39 weeks	Mean 2.30+3SD 3.02	Mean 7.42+3SD 8.71	Mean 5.09+3SD 6.06
40–41 weeks	Mean 2.28+3SD 3.09	Mean 7.35+3SD 8.73	Mean 5.07+3SD 6.30
42–43 weeks	Mean 2.28+3SD 2.88	Mean 7.17+3SD 7.47	Mean 4.89+3SD 5.49

[*]Stimulus intensity is 60 dB above adult threshold, stimulus frequency is 10/sec.

those with apnea have a V-1 interpeak interval of 5.63 ms or longer. Differences in conduction time between newborns of the same conceptional age are considerable and a single study is rarely useful for a diagnosis of brainstem injury. The V-1 interpeak interval continues to decline throughout infancy and attains the adult level at about 1 year.

BAER Audiometry

One important application of BAER technology is the testing of hearing in the newborn. The initial test uses a stimulus intensity of 70 dB. Lack of wave V indicates a hearing loss, and requires repeated tests at higher intensities until obtaining a response threshold (Despland and Galambos, 1980; Mjoen et al., 1982). If wave V is present, the test should be repeated at sequential reductions of 10 dB until the lowest intensity capable of producing wave V is proportional to the intensity of the stimulus, a latency-intensity curve can be drawn, with latency on the Y axis and intensity on the X axis. In normal term newborns, the latency of wave V will decrease by 0.24 to 0.44 ms for each 10 dB increase in sound intensity between 70 and 110 dB.

Among 667 newborns from an intensive care nursery, 11.8% failed to demonstrate wave V at a stimulus intensity of 30 dB and 6.1% failed at 45 dB (Kramer et al., 1989). Almost 50% of newborns who failed the initial test returned for further study one or two months later. Forty-three percent of infants who failed at 45 dB and 73% of infants who failed at 30 dB were hearing impaired. BAER screening in the intensive care nursery is therefore an effective method for detecting future hearing loss.

Conductive Hearing Loss

Transitory conductive hearing losses are common in prematures. However, BAER evidence of a conductive hearing loss that persists on two or more studies at least 2 weeks apart places the newborn at risk for chronic serous otitis media. Such newborns require careful follow-up for hearing loss during infancy (Stockard et al., 1983).

In a conductive hearing loss, the time required to transmit sound across the middle ear and activate the cochlea is prolonged. A reduced total amount of sound energy reaches the cochlea. Consequently, the latency of wave I is prolonged and the latency-intensity curve of wave V shifts to the right by an amount equivalent to the hearing loss, without any alteration in the slope of the curve. Because the latency of wave I is prolonged more than the latency of wave V, the V-I interpeak interval is shortened.

Sensory-Neural Hearing Loss

Sensorineural hearing loss is much less common in newborns than is conductive hearing loss. It occurs most often in newborns who sustained asphyxia or intracranial injury. Brain damage frequently is present as well (Stockard et al., 1983).

Because the cochlea, the auditory nerve, or both are damaged, wave I is either absent or has an elevated threshold. The latency of wave I may be normal or prolonged. If prolonged, the V-I interpeak interval is shortened unless there is intrinsic damage to the brainstem as well. The latency–intensity curve of wave V shifts to the right because of the hearing loss but, unlike the shift seen in conductive hearing loss, the slope of the curve becomes steep – exceeding 0.55 ms/dB.

Disturbances of Brainstem Function

The auditory pathways distribute widely in the brainstem from the lateral medulla to the medial midbrain. Processes that damage the brainstem would not spare the auditory system, and consequently the BAER. The two recognized abnormalities of central processing are (1) prolongation of the V-I interpeak interval and (2) reduction in the amplitude (or absence) of wave V as compared with wave I. BAER recordings can predict cranial ultrasound abnormalities in 82% of patients; BAER abnormalities that correlate with neuroimaging include wave I latency and the III-V interwave latency (Karmel et al., 1988). Even at 5 years of age, the BAER maintains a high specificity and positive predictive value using standardized tests of intelligence, visual-motor, and gross motor function (Majnemer and Rosenblatt, 2000).

Prolongation of the V-I Interpeak Interval   The V-I interpeak interval is prolonged when it exceeds three standard deviations. Among prematures, the V-I interpeak interval declines each week and there is considerable variation among prematures of the same gestational age. For these reasons, the diagnosis of V-I interpeak interval prolongation in prematures should not be attempted.

In term newborns, prolongation of the V-I interpeak interval, is usually associated with severe HIE but also occurs with severe hyperbilirubinemia, some congenital malformations, and metabolic disorders. The significance of interpeak interval prolongation as an indication of brainstem dysfunction increases when associated with a reduction in the V/I amplitude ratio.

Reduction in the V/I Amplitude Ratio   Since waves IV and V appear often as a single wave, the term IV-V/I ratio appears in many studies. This section uses the V/I ratio to include IV-V/I when IV and V are inseparable. When wave I is present, the absence of wave V or a reduction in its amplitude to less than 50% of the amplitude of wave I indicates an extremely unfavorable outcome in high-risk newborns (Hecox et al., 1981; Stockard et al., 1983). Approximately one-third die and survivors have severe neurological damage and hearing loss.

The inferior colliculus generates wave V. Severe total asphyxia specifically damaged this nucleus (see Ch. 4). This group comprises the largest number of newborns with reduced amplitude or absence of wave V.

Visual Evoked Response (VER)

Methods

In measuring the visual evoked response (VER), electrodes are fixed to the vertex (Cz), forehead (Fz), and mid-occipital region (Oz) using electrode paste and gauze squares. The occipital electrode is active, the vertex electrode is referential, and the forehead electrode is a ground. This montage displays positive waves as an upward deflection. Inter-electrode impedances are less than 2000 ohms.

Fixation on a checkerboard with alternating pattern reversal produces an optimal VER. This method is not possible in the newborn, and instead, flash stimulation with a strobe unit is used. Many technical and subject variables profoundly affect the flash VER, and response variability is to be expected. Head position must be consistent with respect to the light source. One-hundred flashes at a rate of 2 c/sec and with the light source 25 cm from the subject are the presented stimulus.

Maturation of the VER

The optimal normal flash VER recorded from the term newborn has five components. The initial low-amplitude initial negative wave has a mean latency of 85 ms. Following the first positive wave, with a latency of 125 ms is a higher amplitude second positive wave at a latency of 195 ms. The second negative wave has a latency of 335 ms, and the final positive wave has a latency of 545 ms (Kurtzberg, 1982). However, the morphology of the VER is variable from day to day and even within the same recording system (Pryds et al., 1988). The morphology is especially variable during wakefulness and active sleep and does not become relatively constant even during quiet sleep until 3 months. Among the five components, the first and third positive waves are frequently absent, and only the major positive deflection is sufficiently constant to have clinical application.

In prematures less than 30 weeks' conceptional age, only a slow negative wave with peak latency greater than 350 ms displays. After 30 weeks, this slow negative wave disappears, replaced by the major positive wave. Initially, this wave has a peak latency of 300 ms. The latency declines in a linear fashion at a rate of 10 ms/week.

Abnormalities of the VER

Three VER abnormalities have been recognized in newborns: (1) atypical morphology due to absence or amplitude reduction of major components; (2) significant hemispheric asymmetry in either morphology or amplitude; and (3) an immature response.

Predicting periventricular leukomalacia was potentially the greatest clinical usefulness of the VER. The geniculocalcarine tract passes through the periventricular white matter and rarely spared in ischemic injury to that region (see Ch. 4).

However, advances in imaging technology have increased the accuracy and specificity of diagnosing periventricular leukomalacia beyond what the expectations of VER. Those infants with normal VER have normal cranial ultrasound findings (Kato et al., 2005; Taylor, 1988; Taylor et al., 1992).

In a study of 79 very low birthweight newborns at 40 weeks conceptional age, 40 had a normal VER, 14 had hemispheric asymmetries (8 in morphology, 6 in amplitude), 19 had an immature response, and 6 had atypical morphology (Kurtzberg, 1982). CT scans showed 24% were abnormal. Periventricular low density (leukomalacia) was present in 92% of newborns with hemispheric asymmetry, 100% with an immature response, and 80% with atypical morphology. Among this group of high-risk newborns, 54% of those with a normal VER were neurologically normal at 1 year. By contrast, only 17% of those with an abnormal VER were neurologically normal at one year. In a study of 54 infants with 2-year follow-up, Taylor et al. (1992) found all those with an absent or abnormal VER throughout the first week of life either died or had severe neurological sequelae (positive predictive value of 100%). At two-year follow-up, no false-positives and 11% false-positives were found with the best prognostic reliability in moderate HIE.

Somatosensory Evoked Response (SSER)

Methods

The maturation of the peripheral nerve and posterior columns progress more rapidly than lemniscal and thalamocortical segments of the somatosensory pathway (Boor and Goebel, 2000). Measurement of the somatosensory evoked response (SSER) involves repetitive electrical stimulation of the median nerve at a rate of 4 c/s and duration of 200 μs at intensity just sufficient to produce a twitch of the thumb. Active electrodes are at Erb's point, over the second cervical spine, and 2 cm behind C3 and C4 on the scalp. Fz is the reference electrode. A negative wave evokes at Erb's point and at the cervical spine in all newborns and at the scalp in 85% (Majnemer et al., 1987). The negative wave (N1) at the scalp has a normal latency of 25 and 30 ms, and followed 5 ms later by a positive wave at 40 weeks. The N1 cortical response is measurable at 28 weeks' gestation (latency 114 ms) which progressively shortens to 71 ms at 31–32 weeks followed by a linear decrease from 31 to 42 weeks of −3.3 ms/week (Karniski et al., 1992; Taylor et al., 1996; Pike et al., 1997).

Abnormalities of the SSER

The predictive value of SSER is of interest since the parietal lobe generators of these waves are in close proximity to the motor cortex and the periventricular white matter region. In larger studies of term infants, increased latency and decreased amplitude of the negative wave at the scalp are noted in asphyxiated newborns and correlate with poor motor cognitive outcome (Majnemer et al., 1987; Willis et al., 1987; Taylor et al., 1992; Majnemer and Rosenblatt, 2000) with a sensitivity of 95–100% and specificity 88%. The use of SSEP in preterm infants and correlation with cranial ultrasound results and developmental outcome is unclear at this time.

REFERENCES AND FURTHER READING

Anders T, Emde R and Parmelee A. A Manual of Standardized Terminology, Techniques and Criteria for Scoring of States of Sleep and Wakefulness in Newborn Infants. UCLA Brain Information Service/ BRI Publications Office. Los Angeles, 1971.

Aso K, Abdab-Barmada M and Scher MS. EEG and the neuropathology in premature neonates with intraventricular hemorrhage. J Clin Neurophysiol 1993;10:304–313.

Aso K, Scher MS and Barmada MA. Neonatal electroencephalography and neuropathology. J Clin Neurophysiol 1989;6:103–123.

Baud O, d'Allest AM, Lacaze-Masmonteil T, et al. The early diagnosis of periventricular leukomalacia in premature infants with positive rolandic sharp waves on serial electroencephalography. J Pediatr 1998;132:813–817.

Benda GI, Engel RC and Zhang YP. Prolonged inactive phases during the discontinuous pattern of prematurity in the electroencephalogram of very-low-birthweight infants. Electroencephalogr Clin Neurophysiol 1989;72:189–197.

Biagioni E, Bartalena L, Biver P, et al. Electroencephalographic dysmaturity in preterm infants: A prognostic tool in the early postnatal period. Neuropediatrics 1996;27:311–316.

Blume WT and Dreyfus-Brisac C. Positive rolandic sharp waves in neonatal EEG; types and significance. Electroencephalogr Clin Neurophysiol 1982;53:277–282.

Boor R and Goebel B. Maturation of near-field and far-field somatosensory evoked potentials after median nerve stimulation in children under 4 years of age. Clin Neurophysiol 2000;111:1070–1081.

Clancy RR, Bergqvist AGC, Dlugos DJ. Neonatal encephalography. In: Ebersole JS and Pedley TA. Current Practice of Clinical Electroencephalography, 3rd edn. Philadelphia: Lippincott, Williams, Wilkins, 2003; pp. 160–245.

Clancy RR and Legido A. Postnatal epilepsy after EEG-confirmed neonatal seizures. Epilepsia 1991; 32:69–76.

Clancy RR and Tharp BR. Positive rolandic sharp waves in the electroencephalograms of premature neonates with intraventricular hemorrhage. EEG Clin Neurophysiol 1984;57:395–404.

Despland PA and Galambos R. Use of the auditory brainstem responses by prematures and newborn infants. Neuropediatrics 1980;11:99–107.

Fenichel GM, Webster DL and Wong, WKT. Intracranial hemorrhage in the term newborn. Arch Neurol 1983;41:30–34.

Ferrari F, Torricelli A, Giustardi A, et al. Bioelectric brain maturation in fullterm infants and in healthy and pathological preterm infants at term post-menstrual age. Early Hum Dev 1992;28:37–63.

Garcias Da Silva LF, Nunes ML, Da Costa JC. Risk factors for developing epilepsy after neonatal seizures. Pediatr Neurol. 30(4):271–7, 2004.

Grigg-Damberger MM, Coker SB, Halsey CL, et al. Neonatal burst suppression: its developmental significance. Pediatr Neurol 1989;5:84–92.

Hecox KE and Cone B. Prognostic importance of brainstem auditory evoked responses after asphyxia. Neurology 1981;31:1429–1433.

Henderson-Smart DJ, Pettigrew AG and Campbell DJ. Clinical apnea and brainstem neural function in preterm infants. N Engl J Med 1983;308:353–357.

Holmes GL and Lombroso CT. Prognostic value of background patterns in the neonatal EEG. J Clin Neurophysiol 1993;10:323–352.

Holmes GL, Logan WJ, Kirkpatrick BV, et al. Central nervous system maturation in the stressed premature. Ann Neurol 1979;6:518–522.

Holmes GL, Rowe J, Hafford J, et al. Prognostic value of the electroencephalogram in neonatal asphyxia. EEG Clin Neurophysiol 1982;53:60–72.

Holst M, Eswaran H, Lowery C, et al. Development of auditory evoked fields in human fetuses and newborns: a longitudinal MEG study. Clin Neurophysiol 2005;116:1949–1955.

Joseph JP, Lesevre N, Dreyfus-Brisac C. Spatio-temporal organization of EEG in premature infants and full-term newborns. EEG Clin Neurophysiol 1976;40:153–168.

Karmel BZ, Gardner JM, Zappulla RA, et al. Brain-stem auditory evoked responses as indicators of early brain insult. Electroencephalogr Clin Neurophysiol 1988;71:429–442.

Karniski W, Wyble L, Lease L, Blair RC. The late somatosensory evoked potential in premature and term infants. II. Topography and latency development. Electroencephalogr Clin Neurophysiol 1992; 84:44–54.

Kato T, Okumura A, Hayakawa F et al. The evolutionary change of flash visual evoked potentials in preterm infants with periventricular leukomalacia. Clin Neurophysiol 2005;116:690–695.

Knauss TA and Carlson CB. Neonatal paroxysmal monorhythmic alpha activity. Arch Neurol 1978;35:104–107.

Kramer SJ, Vertes DR and Condon M. Auditory brainstem responses and clinical follow-up of high-risk infants. Pediatrics 1989;83:385–392.

Kurtzberg D. Event-related potentials in the evaluation of high-risk infants. Ann NY Acad Sci 1982;388:557–571.

Lacey DJ, Topper WH, Buckwald S, et al. Preterm very-low-birth-weight neonates: Relationship of EEG to intracranial hemorrhage, perinatal complications, and developmental outcome. Neurology 1986;36:1084–1087.

Lombroso CT. Some aspects of EEG polygraphy in newborns at risk from neurological disorders. In: PA Buser, WA Cobb, T Okuma (eds). Kyoto Symposia (EEG Suppl. No. 36). Amsterdam: Elsevier Biomedical Press, 1982; pp. 652–653.

Majnemer A and Rosenblatt B. Prediction of outcome at school age in neonatal intensive care unit graduates using neonatal neurologic tools. J Child Neurol 2000;15:645–651.

Majnemer A, Rosenblatt B, Riley P, et al. Somatosensory evoked response abnormalities in high-risk newborns. Pediatr Neurol 1987;3:350–355.

Markand ON, Garg BP, Brandt IK. Nonketotic hyperglycinemia: Electroencephalographic and evoked potential abnormalities. Neurology 1982;32:151–156.

Marret S, Parain D, Jeannot E, et al. Positive rolandic sharp waves in the EEG of the premature newborn: a five year prospective study. Arch Dis Child 1992;67: 948–951.

McCutchen CB, Coen R and Iragui VJ. Periodic lateralized epileptiform discharges in asphyxiated neonates. EEG Clin Neurophysiol 1985;61:210–217.

Mizrahi, EM, Hrachovy, RA, and Kellaway, P. Atlas of Neonatal Electroencephalography, 3rd edn. Philadelphia: Lippincott, Williams and Wilkins, 2003; pp. 55–91.

Mizrahi EM, Pollack MA and Kellaway P. Neocortical death in infants: behavioral, neurologic, and electroencephalographic characteristics. Pediatr Neurol 1985;1:302–305.

Mjoen S, Langslet A, Tangsrud SE, et al. Auditory brainstem responses (ABR) in high-risk neonates. Acta Paediatr Scand 1982;71:711–715.

Nunes ML, Giraldes MM, Pinho AP and Costa JC. Prognostic value of non-reactive burst suppression EEG pattern associated to early neonatal seizures. Arq Neuropsiquiatr 2005;63:14–19.

O'Brien MJ, Lems YL and Prechtl HF. Transient flattenings in the EEG of newborns – a benign variation. Electroencephalogr Clin Neurophysiol 1987;67:16–26.

Ortibus EL, Sum JM and Hahn JS. Predictive value of EEG for outcome and epilepsy following neonatal seizures. Electroencephalogr Clin Neurophysiol 1996;98:175–185.

Osredkar D, Toet MC, van Rooij LG, et al. Sleep-wake cycling on amplitude-integrated electroencephalography in term newborns with hypoxic-ischemic encephalopathy. Pediatrics 2005;115: 327–332.

Parmelee AH, Schulte FJ, Akiyama Y, et al. Maturation of EEG activity during sleep in premature infants. EEG Clin Neurophysiol 1968;24:319–329.

Patrizi S, Holmes GL, Orzalesi M and Allemand F. Neonatal seizures: characteristics of EEG ictal activity in preterm and fullterm infants. Brain Dev 2003;25(6):427–437.

Pike AA, Marlow N and Dawson C. Posterior tibial somatosensory evoked potentials in very preterm infants. Early Hum Dev 1997;47:71–84.

Pryds O, Greisen G and Trojaborg W. Visual evoked potentials in preterm infants during the first hours of life. EEG Clin Neurophysiol 1988;71:257–265.

Salamy A, Eldredge L and Wakeley A. Maturation of contralateral brain-stem responses in preterm infants. EEG Clin Neurophysiol 1985;62:117–123.

Scher MS, Aso K, Beggarly ME, et al. Electrographic seizures in preterm and full-term neonates: clinical correlates, associated brain lesions, and risk for neurologic sequelae. Pediatrics 1993;91:128–134.

Scher MS and Beggarly M. Clinical significance of focal periodic discharges in neonates. J Child Neurol 1989;4:175–185.

Selton D, Andre M and Hascoet JM. Normal EEG in very premature infants: Reference criteria. Clin Neurophysiol 2000;111:2116–1124.

Statz A, Dumermuth G and Mieth D. Transient EEG patterns during sleep in healthy newborns. Neuropediatrics 1982;13:115–122.

Stockard JE, Stockard JJ, Kleinberg F, et al. Prognostic value of brainstem auditory evoked potentials in neonates. Arch Neurol 1983;40:360–365.

Taylor, MJ. Developmental changes in ERPs to visual language stimuli. Biol Psychol 1988;26:321–338.

Taylor MJ, Boor R, Keenan NK, et al. Brainstem auditory and visual evoked potentials in infants with myelomeningocele. Brain Dev 1996;18:99–104.

Taylor MJ, Murphy WJ and Whyte HE. Prognostic reliability of somatosensory and visual evoked potentials of asphyxiated term infants. Dev Med Child Neurol 1992;34:507–515.

Tharp BR, Cukier F and Monod N. The prognostic value of the electroencephalogram in premature infants. EEG Clin Neurophysiol 1981;51:219–235.

Vecchierini-Blineau MF, Nogues B, Louvet S, et al. Positive temporal sharp waves in electroencephalograms of the premature newborn. Neurophysiol Clin 1996;26:350–362.

Vles JSH, Casaer P, Klingma H, et al. A longitudinal study of brainstem auditory evoked potentials of preterm infants. Dev Med Child Neurol 1987;29:577–585.

Watanabe K, Miyazaki S, Hara K, et al. Behavioral state cycles, background EEGs and prognosis of newborns with perinatal hypoxia. EEG Clin Neurophysiol 1980;49:618–625.

Werner SS, Stockard JE and Bickford RG. Atlas of Neonatal Electroencephalography New York: Raven Press, 1977.

Willis J, Duncan C and Bell R. Short-latency somatosensory evoked potentials in perinatal asphyxia. Pediatr Neurol 1987;3:203–207.

Wilson PC, Philpott RH, Spies S, et al. The effect of fetal head compression and fetal acidaemia during labor on human fetal cerebral function as measured by the fetal electroencephalogram. Br J Obstet Gynaecol 1979;86:269–277.

INDEX